# THE
# WEEKEND
# MAKEOVER

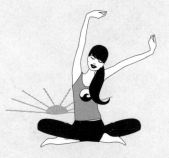

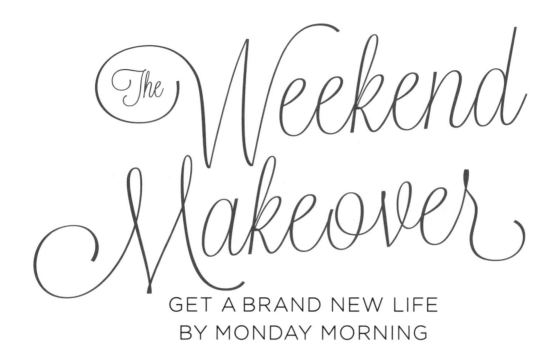

# The Weekend Makeover

## GET A BRAND NEW LIFE BY MONDAY MORNING

Jill Martin & Dana Ravich

RODALE.

© 2013 by Jill Martin and Dana Ravich

Rodale books may be purchased for business or promotional use or for special sales.
For information, please write to:
Special Markets Department, Rodale Inc., 733 Third Avenue, New York, NY 10017.

Printed in the United States of America
Rodale Inc. makes every effort to use acid-free ♾, recycled paper ♲.

Book design by Christina Gaugler
Illustrations by Sydney VanDyke

Library of Congress Cataloging-in-Publication Data is on file with the publisher.
ISBN-13: 978-1-60961-495-9   hardcover

Distributed to the trade by Macmillan
2   4   6   8   10   9   7   5   3   1   hardcover

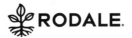

We inspire and enable people to improve their lives and the world around them.
rodalebooks.com

To our families—
all of whom are inspirational throughout these pages—
one way or another!!

Georgette, Marty, Jonathan, Bella,
Lucy, Robert, Helen, Rachel, Lyle, Lou Lou, Leo, Danny—
thank you for your lessons, encouragement,
and most of all your love.

# Contents

# INTRODUCTION

*"I don't have time. I don't have energy.*
*I have a family to take care of. I'm too busy with work.*
*It's too overwhelming. I'm going to start on Monday."*

Sound familiar? We've heard all those excuses before. (Truth be told, we've used a few ourselves from time to time.) No more excuses! It's time for a new program—one that will get you motivated, organized, and on the road to a fabulous and confident new you!

Facing an overhaul in any area of your life can be daunting, and we want you to be successful. So for each chapter of this book, we ask for one weekend. One weekend—just 48 hours—to make a significant change in your diet, your closet, your relationships, even your vacation plans. Can you give us that? Can you give *yourself* that?

The reason we designed this book as a series of "weekend makeovers" is simple. First, a weekend is a block of time that, with a little planning, can be set aside for a single purpose. It is rare that you ever get a moment during the week, let alone a decent chunk of time, to focus on anything other than work, family, and, well, life. Things are usually calmer and quieter over the weekend, allowing you to focus on realistically putting new goals in motion. Weekends are also less disruptive to the rest of the people in your life. This makes it much easier to set aside your regular responsibilities without feeling guilt! Remember: A weekend makeover is not time "off"; it's time well spent to improve your life.

If you are single or living on your own, it may be fairly easy to block out an entire weekend. If you are married with kids, guess what? You still need to take care of *you*. Sure, it requires a little planning to arrange for your husband to schedule his own activities or to organize extra playdates for the kids or a weekend at Grandma and Grandpa's—but clearing your house will give you the necessary space to focus on the task at hand. (We're guessing your husband probably won't mind being asked to spend the day out golfing!) Start getting into the mind-set that you deserve this solo time—we have a feeling that most often you're taking care of everyone else, right?

So, single or married, kids or no kids, whatever your situation, the first step is allowing yourself to allot a weekend (guilt free!) for self-improvement. And believe us, if you have a partner and kids, they will thank you for it. You'll be amazed at how a happier, healthier you makes for a happier, healthier household. You know how when you're listening to safety instructions on an airplane, the flight attendants tell you to put your oxygen mask on first? Same thing here.

In each chapter, we teach you how to make over a different area of your life. You'll learn how to jump-start each makeover with projects that you can complete over the course of one weekend. You'll also learn how to incorporate useful, practical tools that will keep you on the road to success throughout the week and for the rest of your life!

You deserve to have a healthy and fit body, a clear and calm mind, a clutter-free and relaxing home, and a fulfilling social, family, and romantic life. And you can get there, one weekend at a time! You can read the chapters in order if you'd like, or pick the most important or urgent area for change and tackle that topic first. You will see, though, as you finish the makeovers (especially if you follow the chapters in order), that there is overlap in the practice and time commitment. This makes it easier to build on previous makeovers and supports your efforts by giving you confidence and motivation as you go. By the time you've completed all 12 chapters, you will have given yourself a completely new start to a life where you can grow, flourish, and enjoy every moment!

Are you ready? Ready to commit? Ready to change? Ready to be the happiest, healthiest, best you possible? We thought so. Let's get started!

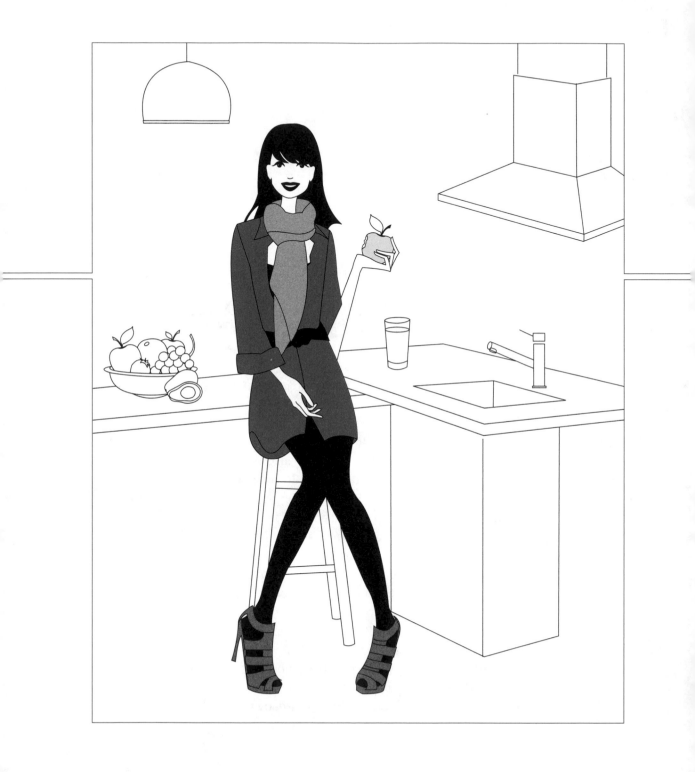

# Chapter One

## Diet Makeover

Do you wish you could lose those last 5 pounds? Do you wish your kids ate healthier foods? Are you overwhelmed by the terms "gluten free," "organic," and "cholesterol free"? Whatever your reasons for wanting to make a change, we could all use an overhaul in the diet department!

It's easy to fall into an eating rut—whatever's fast, whatever's easy, whatever's in the cabinet or fridge. Unfortunately, this pattern can lead to seriously unhealthy habits for you and your family. One study found that availability—or having certain foods in the house—affects what children eat. That's why it's especially important to keep fresh fruits and veggies stocked for kids, even those who already prefer the taste of chips and cookies. Telling kids they can't have junk food while keeping the bad stuff in sight doesn't solve the problem! The good news is that with a little jump start, you and your family will be on the road to better eating habits. By setting a good example and keeping a junk food-free kitchen, you can begin to change your entire household. You will have to be the one to make the decision, take charge, and implement the changes, but once that's all in motion, you can support each other every day with delicious and healthy food choices.

You will need time this weekend to clean out the kitchen, go grocery shopping, and do some cooking. This might not sound too far off from your typical weekend, but we want you to look at this makeover as a fun adventure, not as your usual chores. This Saturday and Sunday, commit to eating foods you prepare yourself at home. (No, microwaving does not count as cooking!) It will be much easier to get on nutritional track without the distractions of restaurants and watching other people eating foods you are trying to avoid. (And, yes, this includes skipping Starbucks, too!)

If you live alone, invite a friend to join you for any or all meals. If you have a partner and/or kids, invite them to join you in eating healthy this weekend and beyond. This makeover isn't about deprivation—it's about doing something rewarding for yourself. By the end of the next 48 hours, you'll have a new attitude toward eating right. It's going to be great, so let's get started!

## ☾ FRIDAY NIGHT

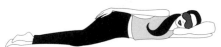

Set the stage for the weekend by relaxing at home with a healthy dinner—whether that means preparing something yourself (if you have the proper groceries) or picking up something healthy on the way home from work (we understand that Friday nights can be tough, timewise, to cook). This is not an excuse to indulge in your last unhealthy meal (pizza and french fries)! Your weekend makeover starts now—savor your first taste of good health!

Once you are sated and the table has been cleared, the fun begins. Do you know the saying "Never go food shopping on an empty stomach"? Well, never clean out your kitchen when you're hungry, either. You don't want to be tempted to snack on items that are on their way to the trash bin. One last cookie, one piece of candy—you get the idea . . . no!

The ultimate goal is to have a clean, organized kitchen full of healthy meal and snack options. To achieve this, you need to purge your kitchen of all the junk. You won't be tempted by what isn't there, right? This means being hard-core about what needs to go. Don't worry, we'll get you on track and walk you through the process.

The most important guideline to follow in revamping your kitchen and your diet is this: Stick to what's all natural. Look for foods that are closest to their natural state; in other words, whole foods (fruits, veggies, and whole grains). Avoid foods that are heavily processed from their original state and therefore devoid of most nutrients—including anything made from white flour (breads and pastas), meats such as hot dogs, and anything containing a ton of added salt and/or sugar.

In addition, buying organic when possible can be a plus. Organically grown foods typically contain none of the chemical pesticides of commercially grown foods—although one recent study claims that there is no nutritional difference between organic and conventional food, which is good news for your wallet if organic food is more expensive in your neighborhood.

If you have a dietary restriction, such as gluten sensitivity or lactose intolerance, note which foods you should avoid and purge your kitchen of those culprits now. If you have specific health concerns, such as high blood pressure or high cholesterol, you may want to think about reducing or eliminating meat (especially red meat) from your diet.

**Start with the fridge.** Anything past its expiration date must go. Even so-called healthy staples go bad, so look at everything in the fridge. Yes, everything! Old dairy products that may have curdled, leftover meat from you can't remember when, fruit that has mold, or other lettuce or veggies with brown spots: Toss 'em.

## TOP 10 CONDIMENTS' SHELF LIFE, ONCE OPENED

1. Butter: 3 months in fridge
2. Chili sauce: 1 month in pantry, longer in fridge
3. Jelly/jam: 1 year in fridge
4. Ketchup: 1 month in pantry, a bit longer in fridge
5. Mayonnaise: 2 months in fridge
6. Mustard: 6–8 months in pantry or fridge
7. Peanut butter: 2–3 months in pantry, longer in fridge
8. Salad dressing: 3 months in fridge
9. Sour cream: 2 weeks in fridge
10. Vegetable oil: 1–3 months, best stored in fridge

*Jill*

*My mother needs to skip this paragraph. (Mom, if you are reading this, move on to Dana's story!) Here's the deal: My mama isn't a great cook. Well, wait. I shouldn't say that. She says she can make the best French onion soup on the planet (however, my brother and I have never had it!), and she does make delicious chocolate chip pancakes. Needless to say, she is the best mom in the world. But like many of us, I grew up eating a lot of pizza and takeout. Since turning 35, my body has changed, and I can't, unfortunately, eat whatever I want whenever I want. If I were to splurge on even an order of fries now, I would feel it. (Ladies, I know you can relate.) So I have to be creative and look for ways to snack without gaining weight. My first rule is that I never keep anything I love too much in the house. I can't eat just one cookie. . . . I eat the whole box. My second rule is to always ask other people for their tricks. Today nutritionist Joy Bauer taught me a potion that helps keep me out of snack trouble: Mix a plain Greek yogurt with a pack of sugar-free hot cocoa. Voilà—chocolate pudding! It is nutritious, fills me up, and satisfies my sweet tooth.*

*Dana*

*I am very good about not wasting food. I know exactly how much I need and what I will and won't eat, so I never keep extra stuff in the fridge that could go bad. I always have everything I need for a snack or an actual meal. (Full disclaimer: I am a raw vegan, so all I have are fruits, veggies, nuts and seeds, and some raw dessert treats. Oh, and a freezer full of coconut water, but that's a whole other story!) Regardless of what's in there, my fridge and freezer are organized, and there is nothing old, rotten, moldy, or unidentifiable. However, when I visit my sister, I have a field day. As soon as I get to her house, I go straight to the fridge and start looking through containers, opening them, smelling things, and throwing things away. I think it drives her nuts (sorry, Sis!), but I can't stand having that old stuff in there and can't bear to ask if the kale is from the last time I visited.*

Anything else that hasn't spoiled but that you know is bad for you (pudding, cake, cookies) has to go, too. This includes processed foods that have been in the fridge for a while: If they haven't spoiled, that probably means they are made of, or preserved with, a ton of chemicals. Either way, processed food qualifies as "junk" and therefore goes in the garbage.

Don't forget to examine the condiments, too. We tend to overlook those random bottles and jars on the refrigerator door. For some reason, we think these products will last forever. Cleaning out the fridge door is the perfect opportunity to start fresh and start healthy. So unless you're holding a recently purchased jar of quality mustard (think Grey Poupon, not French's) or a brand-new all-fruit jam, you probably want to toss that condiment.

Don't be afraid to really purge. It's okay if your fridge looks barren—you just had a healthy, satisfying dinner, and tomorrow you are going to fill the refrigerator with all the right foods. If an empty fridge truly bothers you, think of this process as preparing to go on vacation: You wouldn't want to leave anything to spoil while you are out of town.

**Move on to the freezer.** If you think your fridge door was a mess, the freezer can be a vast wasteland of forgotten items. Even though frozen foods essentially last forever, over time they do lose quality and taste.

Toss anything that has freezer burn and anything you haven't used in the past 3 to 6 months. While freezing food can be a great way to preserve it, that old turkey burger with frostbite isn't exactly an appealing dinner option. When and if you need a bag of frozen peas, you can pop to the store—or better yet, buy fresh peas. In addition, get rid of all the ice cream, sugary ice pops, and frozen desserts that are laden with sugar and fat. (If you find yourself hesitating, simply add up all the calories from each box and you'll be eager not to have them around!)

> # TOP 10 FROZEN ESSENTIALS' SHELF LIFE
>
> 1. Butter: 9 months
> 2. Fish: 3–6 months
> 3. Fruits/berries: 8–12 months
> 4. Grains: 4 months
> 5. Lean meats: 6 months
> 6. Nuts: 2 years
> 7. Sauces: 6 months
> 8. Seeds: 2 years
> 9. Soups: 6 months
> 10. Veggies: 8–12 months

**Get into your cabinets and pantry.** Dry goods must also be inspected. Check the age of your cereal. Have any boxes been left open? It's important to keep boxes of cereal and other dry grains airtight. If dry goods haven't been tightly sealed, or you can't remember when you bought them, toss them and start fresh. Now, about those cookies, crackers, chips, roasted nuts, and candy . . . junk, junk, and junk! We think you know what to do with these by now—that's right, dump 'em. (Thank you.)

Artificial sweeteners? Table salt? Refined sugar? Those can definitely go, too. And about the spices, teas, and oils—if you use them in your cooking, great; they can stay. But organize them in your cabinet, either by height with stacking racks or in clearly labeled containers, so you can quickly find the one you need. Your goal is to have a clean, fully functioning kitchen that you can restock with healthy items tomorrow.

Congrats—you are finished for the evening! You should feel lighter already and very proud of yourself for letting go of all the junk. Tomorrow will be an adventure in grocery shopping!

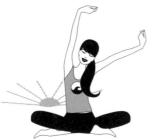

# SATURDAY MORNING

As we mentioned, you don't want to shop for groceries on an empty stomach, or you will crave everything in sight! Take the time to have a healthy and nourishing breakfast—perhaps some fresh fruit, Greek yogurt, oatmeal, or a smoothie. We know we asked you to trash practically everything in the kitchen last night, and hopefully you salvaged something healthy for breakfast. If that's not the case, then go someplace where you can get a healthy, yummy meal before you start grocery shopping.

If you enjoy tea or coffee in the morning, by all means relax and have a cup. Just be aware that how you sweeten your hot beverage is another story. As part of your diet makeover, we're asking you to switch to natural sweeteners, like stevia, instead of artificial sweeteners or refined sugar, and to use almond milk or rice milk instead of artificial creamers (organic cow's milk is okay). A small change in your daily routine is a huge step in the right direction for your overall health.

**Make your shopping list.** The following are categories of foods that should be on your grocery list. Many of the specifics within the categories are up to you—we simply recommend filling your kitchen with a range of healthy options. Pick what you like, but branch out into items you may not have tried before. You'll be amazed at the variety in the store and especially at farmers' markets once you take the time to look. You might surprise yourself and find a new favorite!

## Fresh Fruit

Think beyond just apples! Buy fruit that's easy to reach for as a snack (grapes, blueberries, cherries). Buy some that you can use for smoothies (bananas and berries). Buy some to eat for breakfast (cantaloupe, honeydew, watermelon). And don't forget a sweet dessert treat (pineapple and strawberries). There are no rules here. *All* fresh fruit is good for you, so pick your faves! And experiment with more exotic types, like mango, papaya, and persimmon. The more healthy options you have, the more variety you will enjoy and the more satisfied you will be.

## Fresh Veggies

Here, too, you don't have to stick to carrots and celery. A world of delicious vegetables can be used for different snacks and meals. Instead of iceberg lettuce (which has zero nutritional value), try using kale or spinach as a salad base. These are both chock-full of vitamins, minerals, protein, iron, and fiber, not to mention they make delicious side dishes when sautéed with a little olive oil and garlic. You can experiment with baking your own kale chips—a perfect snack. Or make a chopped salad using radishes, carrots, snap peas, cucumbers, bell peppers, and jicama. These are all perfect snacking veggies, too, either plain or dipped in hummus or guacamole. Salad doesn't have to be just lettuce and tomato—although tomatoes are a healthy addition to any meal (and cherry tomatoes make a delicious snack). Sprouts are a good source of protein, fiber, and vitamins. Avocado is a healthy source of fat (and provides nearly 20 essential nutrients), is supersatisfying, will fill you up, and feels as indulgent as cheese or meat in a salad or sandwich. Swap a hearty portobello mushroom for a burger if you're looking to cut back on red meat.

## Fresh and Dried Herbs

Herbs can make any dish go from just okay to sensational—and which you use is a matter of personal taste. Some to try are basil, mint, cilantro, rosemary, thyme, and parsley. These are great in salads, soups, sauces, guacamole, and any meat or fish dish.

Fresh herbs should be stored in the fridge with your veggies. They will wilt and turn yellowish brown after about a week or so, when they are no longer fresh. Dried herbs will last about a year. Keep them away from heat and moisture, preferably in a tightly sealed container.

## Whole Grains

Maybe you already cook with brown rice. But have you ever tried quinoa or millet or even spelt pasta? There are a ton of grains that can broaden your horizons, including oatmeal and whole grain cereals, whole grain breads, and even baked chips. You don't have to give up bread and pasta entirely. Just look for choices with healthy ingredients. Eating whole grains reduces your risk of a host of health issues, including stroke, type 2 diabetes, heart disease, and high blood pressure—and, most noticeably, can help you shed a few pounds! (If you have a gluten sensitivity, take care to buy only gluten-free products.) Whole grains have more nutrients and more fiber than their white flour counterparts, and your body will digest and use these nutrients much more effectively. In contrast, when you eat products made of white flour, your body registers the processed grains as sugar and ends up storing those calories as fat. Not what you wanted? We didn't think so!

## Organic Dairy Products or Nondairy Substitutes

If you are going to eat dairy, please try to make it organic whenever possible. Nonorganic milk and milk products can contain antibiotics and hormones, and you certainly don't want that. If you have a dairy allergy, are lactose intolerant, or prefer to avoid dairy, there are plenty of options: Soy, almond, rice, and even coconut milk are available as milk substitutes, as are products made with these nondairy substitutes. Peruse the dairy and frozen aisles for products that appeal to you—Greek yogurt, perhaps, or soy yogurt, or frozen deserts made from soy or coconut milk. If you are trying to lose weight, though, hold off on the frozen desserts. Even though they might be healthier options than their dairy counter-parts, they will likely still contain some fat and natural sugars. If your goal is simply to eat healthier, indulge in a natural dessert on occasion. Just be sure to read the dessert's ingredient list. Remember, the fewer ingredients, the better.

## Lean Meats, Fish, and Eggs

Perhaps you eat all of the above—or none. The choice is, of course, up to you and what your goals or health concerns are. Consider purchasing free-range eggs (studies show they have more heart-healthy omega-3 fatty acids plus vitamins A and E), grass-fed meats, and wild (not farmed) fish.

Cholesterol is found in animal products, so if you are trying to lower your cholesterol levels, check with your physician first to determine how much, if any, animal protein you can eat. Even if cholesterol isn't a concern, most Americans are heavy-handed on protein and portion size. The recommended amount of daily protein intake in grams is your body weight multiplied by 0.37. Whatever protein source you choose, note that you don't need that much to fill up or to get enough protein. Your best bet is to have a small portion of meat or fish (about 3 ounces, about the size of a deck of cards) and larger portions of salad, veggies, and grains on the side.

## Beans, Tofu, and Tempeh

If you choose not to eat meat or you just want to change up your diet, beans, tofu, and

## 6 REASONS TO EAT ORGANIC GRASS-FED, NOT GRAIN-FED, PROTEIN

1. Fewer calories
2. Lower total fat content
3. More "good" fats—omega-3 fatty acids
4. No added hormones
5. No antibiotics
6. Richer in antioxidants— vitamin E, beta-carotene, and vitamin C

tempeh are fantastic protein sources. Beans can be used in everything from soups to salads to side dishes. (When combined with rice, quinoa, millet, or other grains, they make a complete protein.) Tofu and tempeh can be seasoned to taste however you like. They are great in stir-fries and as a meat substitute for a main course. If you are (or are trying to be) vegetarian or vegan, make sure to switch up your protein choices, as the saying "everything in moderation" applies to soy as well. When you are buying soy products, choose those made from non–genetically modified (non-GMO) soybeans, as genetically modified foods create proteins that are not naturally found in its structure.

## Raw Nuts, Seeds, and Nut Butters

These are great snacks and healthy sources of fat and protein. Studies show that eating nuts can lower your LDL (or "bad" cholesterol) and reduce your risk of heart disease. Eating a very small amount will keep you satisfied and energized between meals. We specifically say *raw* nuts and seeds because that is the healthiest form to consume. Roasted and/or salted nuts are packed with sodium and extra fat and calories—a big no-no! You can choose from a huge variety of nuts and nut butters—almonds, walnuts, cashews, pistachios, macadamia nuts, and Brazil nuts, to name a few. Seeds are a tasty addition to any salad—flaxseeds, pumpkin seeds, sesame seeds, and more. Flaxseed crackers are delicious, full of fiber, and a great alternative to regular crackers and chips when you want something crunchy!

## Condiments: Oils, Spices, Salt, Sweeteners

You will add to this category as you start to cook more adventurously and find new recipes that you like. Definitely purchase a good olive oil—which contains healthy dietary fat and can lower your risk of heart disease—and also try flaxseed oil, sesame oil, and coconut oil. A full, organized spice rack is also handy, so that you have everything your recipe calls for at the ready. And, of course, look for a quality mustard, reduced-sodium soy sauce or tamari, Celtic sea salt, all-natural ketchup, honey, agave syrup, stevia, and pure maple syrup.

**Hit the market.** Now that you know what you're looking for, it's time to go shopping! If it's a beautiful day and you have a farmers' market nearby, go there first and get as much as you can from local vendors. Hitting your local farmers' market will give you the most bang for your produce buck (and the produce will be fresher and will last longer than what you get at the grocery store). This is also a great way to sample items and ask questions about where your food comes from. You'll be amazed how good it feels to shop for your food in the fresh air—such a different experience from the freezing-cold air-conditioned and fluorescent-lit supermarkets. (Treat yourself to some fresh-cut flowers, too. This is sure to put a smile on your face and brighten up your kitchen!)

You should have your shopping list handy and be crossing items off of it, but it's also fun to wander around the farmers' market or explore the aisles of the grocery store to see what is fresh, is in season, and looks appealing. Shop for food the way you would shop for clothing. Browse, sample (of course, only from the healthy food groups on your shopping list!), and get inspired. Take your time. It's when we're really rushed that we forget the things we need. If you want to make the whole experience even more fun, recruit a friend or your husband (if you both can find the time) to go with you. Turn grocery shopping into an enjoyable way to spend the morning, not just a chore.

You might not be able to get everything you need from the farmers' market, although you will be surprised at how much you can purchase there. Every market is different—some are big and comprehensive, selling everything from produce to baked goods to dairy and meat; some sell only fresh produce. If there is anything on your list that you didn't find at the farmers' market, hit a healthy supermarket next. You will be able to fill in the gaps with any condiments, frozen goods, or dry goods. If you choose a specialty grocer such as Trader Joe's or Whole Foods Market, you will find a wide variety of the healthy fare that you are looking for, and the salespeople will likely be knowledgeable about these items and able to help

## 10 FOODS TO KEEP IN THE FRIDGE

1. Grains
2. Jellies/jams
3. Ketchup
4. Mustard
5. Nut butters
6. Nuts ✓
7. Ripe fruit
8. Ripe veggies
9. Seeds
10. Vegetable oils ✓

you find what you need. If you don't have a Trader Joe's, a Whole Foods, or something similar near you, note that most supermarkets are getting better about carrying organic and other more health-conscious items. Look for those aisles (or ask someone in the store to direct you to them).

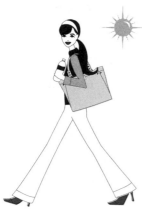

# SATURDAY AFTERNOON

Have everything you need? Yes, it is a lot to carry, but remember, there's no rush. Take your time getting to the car and into the house. You set this weekend aside for this purpose. Your health and well-being are your project for the weekend, so relax and enjoy the process.

**Get organized.** This is your chance to really enjoy going into your kitchen and look forward to what's in there, so don't just toss everything into your newly cleaned fridge! Obviously,

## BOOST NUTRITION AND CUT FAT AND CALORIES

- Before you snack, have a glass of water to make sure you are truly hungry and not just thirsty.
- Use mustard instead of mayo in tuna salad and on sandwiches.
- Use apple slices instead of crackers with everything from cheese to nut butters.
- Use flaxseed oil instead of other oils wherever you can to make sure you get the essential omega-3 and omega-6 fatty acids.
- Purchase pistachios in the shells—they take longer to open and eat than other nuts, so you will eat fewer.
- Have a baked sweet potato instead of fries.
- Never skip breakfast.
- Don't eat after 7:00 p.m.

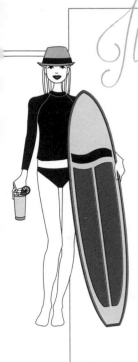

*Jill* *My dream go-to snack? Munchkins from Dunkin' Donuts! Okay, back to reality. I am a huge fan of midday fruit smoothies. I go to a tiny cart in the middle of Union Square in New York City and order a juice to hold me over between meals. But even a juice has calories, so I drink smoothies in moderation. I have one small drink a day, and I opt for it to be made without yogurt. Don't waste all your calories in one shot!*

*Dana* *Fruit is my go-to snack no matter what time of day. It satisfies my sweet tooth, quenches my thirst, and gives me a ton of vitamins. It is also extremely portable. If I am in a hurry or walking around, I go for a fresh-squeezed juice instead. Talk about easy and healthy! My other go-to snacks are raw vegan chocolate macaroons from Pure Food and Wine in New York City. They are delicious and a healthy source of fat. Even if you are trying to lose weight, fat is still a crucial part of any diet.*

if you have frozen items—frozen veggies, whole grain waffles, meat, or fish—they should be put away first. Try to group things in your freezer by category, and make sure you can see everything clearly when you open the door.

Next, take care of the refrigerated items. Put away everything except for the fruit and what you will need to prepare your lunch (we'll explain in a minute). Store nuts and seeds in the fridge, too, as these can go bad when left out. Again, organize everything by category—greens together, veggies together, any dairy or nondairy items together, and so on. Then, when you go to make a salad, or anything else for that matter, the task will be easier—you won't forget anything if you don't have to search around and behind other items.

Then, take care of the pantry or cabinet items. Organize your cereal and your grains nicely so that your cabinets are inviting and easy to manage. You might want to treat yourself to new food storage canisters with labels for your cereals and grains. Place your spices and oils where they look pretty. This will make it so much more appealing when you think about cooking a meal. Next, cut and arrange your fresh flowers. Put some in the kitchen, in the living room, and on your nightstand. These will make you feel happy and relaxed at home and in the kitchen.

## 12 COOKBOOKS, WEB SITES, AND BLOGS WE LOVE

1. *The Art of Simple Food,* by Alice Waters

2. *Cook with Jamie,* by Jamie Oliver

3. *Home Cooking with Jean-Georges,* by Jean-Georges Vongerichten

4. *Joy of Cooking,* by Irma S. Rombauer and Marion Rombauer Becker

5. *The Kind Diet,* by Alicia Silverstone

6. *My Father's Daughter,* by Gwyneth Paltrow

7. *Skinny Bitch: Ultimate Everyday Cookbook,* by Kim Barnouin

8. www.drbenkim.com

9. www.epicurious.com

10. www.foodnetwork.com

11. www.goop.com

12. www.kimberlysnyder.net/blog

Now, why did we wait to put away the fruit? No one grabs for an uncut melon or for unwashed grapes, right? We thought not. Part of this weekend is about creating new habits to help you eat healthy and to make better choices so easy they're impossible to resist!

So, before you put away any of the fruit (except for apples and bananas, which, if you don't grab for those, we can't help you there!), cut it up and store it in sealed containers in the fridge, ready for breakfast, a snack, or dessert or to toss into the blender for a smoothie. Wash the grapes, blueberries, strawberries, raspberries, and any other snackable fruit that just needs a rinse and place them front and center in the fridge, maybe in pretty bowls or in a colander. Think of all the times you want a quick snack or something sweet and you reach for a cookie or a piece of candy. Can you imagine how much healthier—not to mention lighter—you will be when you reach for the fruit instead? Amazing!

Now it's time for lunch. You have a kitchen and pantry full of incredible, fresh, and healthy food at your fingertips. What will you have? A big salad? A veggie sandwich on whole grain bread? A bowl of quinoa with steamed broccoli and kale? Whatever ingredients you choose from your newly revamped kitchen, you are already on the road to a healthier future.

Here's a tip: Eat what interests you. As long as you follow the basic guidelines of what constitutes whole foods, it's good to stay curious and entice yourself with new ideas—or just remind yourself of little ways to add a kick to your diet. Known for their vitamin C and refreshing taste, lemons are ideal squeezed in salad dressings or sliced in your water. A high-quality green powder for your smoothies ups the nutritional value and keeps you satiated. Kelp or dulse flakes are the ultimate salt substitute, as they are packed with tons of minerals and give you that same savory flavor. And how about a little dark chocolate? Yes, now we're talking! You can have your chocolate fix because the dark form is packed with antioxidants.

If you're not good at improvising, keep a few trusty cookbooks on hand and mark the recipes you love. See "12 Cookbooks, Web Sites, and Blogs We Love," opposite.

Congrats! You've already had three healthy meals this weekend, and you are the proud owner of a kitchen full of good-for-you snacks and meal ingredients. Take the rest of the afternoon to do something fun or relaxing (or both) and get your mind off eating for a bit.

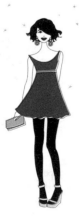

# SATURDAY NIGHT

Now it's time to prepare dinner. Whether you are cooking for yourself or you have invited your partner and/or friends to join you, try something new. Decide what type of cuisine you want to eat and look up a recipe. Maybe you are in the mood for Italian food, and dinner will be spelt pasta with homemade tomato sauce, bruschetta made with a whole grain baguette, and sautéed spinach paired with a nice wine, if you like. Or maybe you want to whip up an Asian-inspired stir-fry with snap peas, mushrooms, carrots, cabbage, and tempeh over brown rice with a side of bok choy. Or you might simply be in the mood for a piece of grilled salmon with steamed asparagus and a baked potato. Totally up to you!

**Take your time.** The trick to eating well is to have fun and make each meal a pleasurable experience. Prepare dinner knowing that you are taking care of yourself and those around you. Take the time to set the table beautifully, even if the meal is just for you. Make it a real dining experience, not a task to be hurried through. Once you view eating as a pleasurable activity and not as a chore or something you don't have time for, you will feel much better.

It takes 20 minutes for your brain to register that your belly feels full. When you eat too quickly, you are more likely to eat too much and not even realize that you've had enough. Slow it down. Other cultures make meals an important part of their day. They have smaller portions, savor their food, enjoy the company they are with, and, as a result, have smaller waistlines, experience less stress, and live longer, healthier lives.

Get in the habit this weekend of truly savoring your food and making eating an event. Don't chow down while you are working, watching TV, or going through the mail. This weekend is all about you. You are on a mini-break, and what you do this

## Jill

*I eat the same thing for breakfast every day, and even I can cook it!* Today *nutritionist Joy Bauer introduced me to Amy's Breakfast Burritos, which I can get at any health food market. All I do is heat one up and add a little salsa, and it is ready to go. These keep me full until lunch, which is very important, as I get up very early for work every day and need something that gets me going and keeps me going until I am off the air at about 11:00 a.m.*

## Dana

*Every day, I start my morning with a green drink concoction I came up with after a few experiments. I mix a heaping tablespoon of spirulina (which I order from Keith Smith's Herb Shop in California) with a heaping tablespoon of high-quality green powder (I use Dr. Ben Kim's Greens, which I order online) in a tall glass of coconut water. This has all the vitamins, minerals, and nutrients I need for the day. I feel great beginning my day this way. This drink and some fresh fruit midmorning keep me totally satiated until lunch.*

weekend will set the tone for how you go back to your everyday life. Enjoy your dinner and, if you've invited people to join you, your company. This is the best kind of Saturday night! Relax, unwind, and eat slowly. Savor every bite, chew your food thoroughly, and notice how much better you feel from these small yet impactful changes. Linger over your meal. When everyone is finished, clean up and return your kitchen to its newly organized and beautiful state. You'll feel happy and refreshed when you walk into an inviting kitchen in the morning. Sleep well.

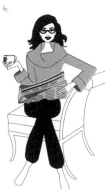

# SUNDAY

When you wake up, prepare a healthy, energizing breakfast. Savor it, whether with company or solo. This weekend is yours, and you have nowhere to rush off to. Take some time to leisurely peruse the newspaper, or to leaf through recipe books or search on the Internet for new recipes to try this coming week.

We don't necessarily expect you to always eat at home and to craft each meal slowly and thoughtfully, but we would like you to commit to preparing a certain number of meals per week for yourself and your loved ones. These meals should be eaten with care—meaning slowly, not while surfing the Internet or watching a movie—and at a beautifully set table. Food researcher Brian Wansink found that some people lost up to 2 pounds a month simply by swapping smaller salad plates for large dinner plates and eating in the kitchen or dining room instead of in front of the TV!

**Make a meal schedule—and stick to it.** Today, decide how many and which meals you'll plan. Make an actual schedule, even if it means writing down the details in your date book. If your days are crazy busy with work, kids, and a ton of other responsibilities, maybe dinner is the meal you can commit to cooking at home. If that's the case, you can plan to make extra helpings of dinner and bring the leftovers to work for lunch the next day. Once you get the hang of eating healthier and more slowly, it will become second nature. A habit only takes 3 weeks (or 21 days, whichever seems more palatable to you!) to form or break.

If you can commit to sticking to your food plan for that period, the foods you used to crave won't seem so appealing anymore, and you will start to notice positive changes. You might feel lighter, you might notice that you have better digestion, you might experience clearer skin or even better sleep.

**Don't skip breakfast!** For the next few weeks, make the extra effort to have a solid breakfast. Whether it means getting up a half hour earlier or sitting down with your kids in the morning instead of rushing to get out of the house, commit to starting your day right. This one step will make your food choices for the rest of the day that much easier and healthier. By keeping your metabolism humming, you won't experience the crash that so often happens when lunchtime rolls around and you're running on empty, ravenously reaching for the easiest, fastest, and probably least healthy option!

**Pack a snack and a lunch.** Take the time today to prepare healthy snacks for between meals, and pack some of them up to take to work in the coming days. Your snacks could be fresh fruit (melon, pineapple, grapes, berries) or fresh-cut veggies (peppers, carrots, celery, cucumber, tomatoes) in a sealed container, a small portion of nuts in a zipper-lock bag, some flaxseed crackers, $\frac{1}{3}$ cup of shelled edamame, or half an avocado. Eating healthy snacks means you'll keep your portion sizes down at meals and help regulate your blood sugar and maintain your energy throughout the day.

If you are able to bring something you've made yourself for lunch at work, great. If not, keep your goals in mind when you go out to grab lunch during the week. Keep food choices healthy and try to take it slowly. It's so easy to get rushed during a crazy day at work or while running the kids around to their activities, and to make bad choices. But take a deep breath whenever you can and try your best to make mealtime your time.

**Customize your kitchen—even if it's not your kitchen.** Of course, we know it's not realistic to expect you to eat every meal at home. However, you are now on the right track to healthy eating all of the time. You have made the commitment to change your eating habits—to choose healthier options for yourself and your family.

Keep tabs on what you eat and what ingredients need to be replaced so you can maintain this sense of order and calm. Perhaps you can make attending the farmers' market part of your ongoing weekend ritual and then pick up other odds and ends at the grocery store during the week or as you need them.

This weekend you've stocked your kitchen with good-for-you meal options. Stick to this commitment when you are deciding what to order in a restaurant. First, choose restaurants that have healthy dishes and farm-to-table experiences, organic food restaurants, or eateries with vegetarian options. (Yes, this means no fast-food joints!) Even if the restaurant choice is not up to you, you can always select one of the healthier options on the menu. Almost every restaurant has a salad or can grill a piece of fish or chicken.

*Restaurants*

Second, don't be afraid to ask for a meal to be prepared according to your preferences. Most restaurants these days will accommodate all types of eaters. Simply ask to have your food grilled instead of fried or served with a lighter sauce—say, a tomato sauce versus one made with heavy cream. Or ask the chef to make you a dish without dairy or gluten.

Then, keep your environment as temptation free as possible. Ask the waiter not to leave the bread basket on the table, if bread is your weakness. Request an appetizer portion if you are worried about controlling how much you eat. And don't look at a dessert menu if you know you'll order the chocolate lava cake and feel terrible afterward!

While you are still relaxing at home today, continue to treat yourself well and take the time to savor your food. Prepare another luxurious dinner this evening, one that introduces the whole family (kids included) to your new and improved eating plan. You'll sleep soundly knowing that, in just 48 hours, you made a significant change in your health and the health of your family—and that you're all on track for a better and brighter future.

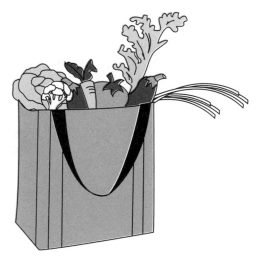

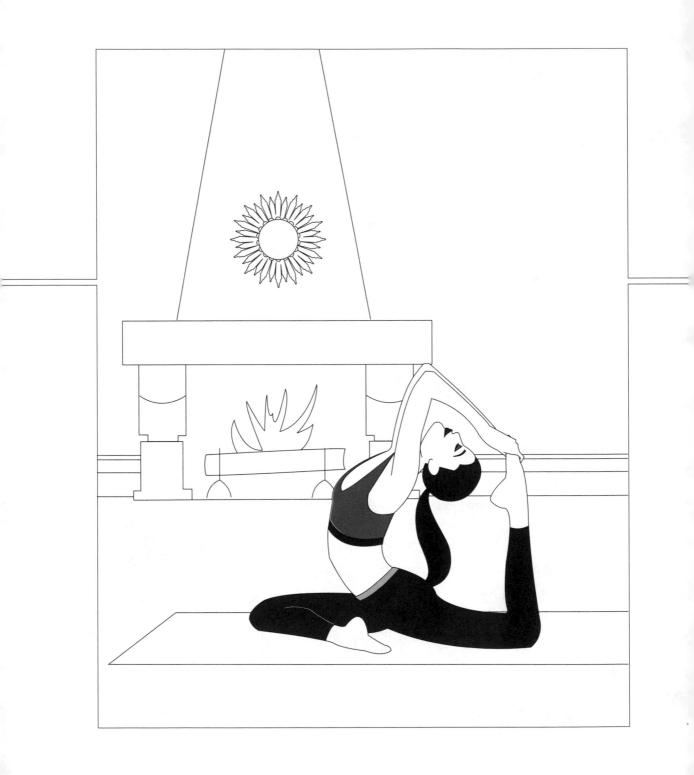

# Chapter Two

# Workout Makeover

Who *doesn't* want a better body—to be more in shape, feel fit and sexy, and look great to boot? No one who we've come across! The number-one thing people would change if they could is the way their body looks. Well, guess what? You *can* change your body! Really, we promise. It just takes a bit of work—let's not even call it work, let's call it a *commitment*. And you can make it fun! The idea is to find a workout that you enjoy and look forward to. We are going to build a routine around something that you love to do *and* that makes you look and feel amazing in one fell swoop!

Can you commit to this? Can you commit to giving yourself a weekend to make this change? One weekend is all you need to get on the road to not only your dream body but also a healthier, more active life! You deserve this. Just like any form of self-improvement, the results of your efforts will be a huge and great change for you and for everyone around you. Your family and loved ones will

## 10 EXERCISES TO GET LEAN

1. Dancing
2. Hiking
3. Jumping rope
4. Power walking
5. Running
6. Skiing
7. Spinning/bicycling
8. Stairclimber/elliptical machine
9. Swimming
10. Tennis

appreciate the new calmer, healthier, happier you—and they may even get inspired to get in shape, too.

Working out, exercising, and playing sports are something you can do alone or with a partner. So even though this weekend is all about finding your path, if you would like to embark on this journey with a partner or friend, that's great. Some people do better when another person pushes them. Perhaps having an obligation to meet up for a workout is enough to ensure you show up. It's all personal preference, so whatever approach you choose is up to you.

Schedule your weekend so you have the time and ability to jump right into your workout makeover. Are you ready? There's no time like the present, so let's get started!

# ☾ FRIDAY NIGHT

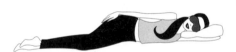

You can become leaner, more toned, stronger, and more flexible and look better in clothes (or a bikini!)—or whatever your goal is. However, we cannot make you taller, shorter, or change the color of your eyes! When you are looking through magazines and coveting the same body as your favorite celeb, please remember that every body is different. Even Jennifer Aniston will never have Gisele Bündchen's body, or vice versa. Both women are in great shape and have fabulous figures, but they're different. So take body type into account and be realistic when you look for fitness inspiration. Don't worry so much about what everybody else looks like; instead, let's figure out how you can look like your best *you*!

**Get inspired.** Relax, enjoy a healthy dinner (a new body depends on smart, healthy eating as much as on a consistent workout routine), and then take time to look through fitness and/or fashion magazines for inspiration. Tear out the pictures of people who make you want to run to the gym right now, then make an inspiration board. This could mean taping a couple of pictures to your fridge or tacking photos to a bulletin board above your desk. Either way, you will have a constant reminder of your goal. And by the way, the pictures could be of yourself from a few years back—perhaps from before you had kids or got too busy to keep doing your workouts. These types of pictures are the best motivation of all, because you know what you are capable of. Got your inspiration? Great! You now have something to work toward.

**Find your routine.** The next step is to find a workout routine that will get you to your goal *and* keep you challenged and enjoying yourself so you'll stay committed as you start seeing results. Keep in mind that if you want to lose weight or get leaner, you will want to focus on cardio (activities like running, biking, hiking, which burns calories by getting your heart rate up for at least 20 minutes) and stretching (which elongates muscles for a leaner appearance). If your goal is to build muscle and get toned, you will want to focus on strength training with weights or resistance (added bonus: maintaining muscle boosts metabolism and burns fat).

Here's the thing: Any and all exercise is good for you. Unless you are lifting heavy weights every day and training like a bodybuilder, you are not going to get too bulky (which we are assuming nobody reading this wants!). Ideally, any workout, along with a healthy diet, will make you both leaner and stronger. The most important thing is to figure out an activity (or a few different ones) that you love so that you will be sure to stick to a routine.

A few things to keep in mind as you choose:

## 10 EXERCISES TO GET TONED

1. Calisthenics/matwork
2. Gymnastics
3. Horseback riding
4. Kettlebells
5. Paddleboarding
6. Pilates
7. Rock climbing
8. Surfing
9. Weight training
10. Yoga

## Where Do You Live?

If you live in a warmer climate, you have the option of exercising outdoors year-round, whereas if you live up north, you will likely need to find an indoor activity for the colder months. If you live someplace mountainous like California, perhaps you prefer hiking outdoors, whereas if you live someplace flat and urban like New York City, you may want to walk on an incline on a treadmill. That said, some people do run outside all year long, no matter what the weather, and some people in hot climates prefer to exercise in an air-conditioned gym. Then, of course, there are indoor pools in cold climates, just as there is indoor rock climbing, indoor ice-skating, and indoor tennis. At the end of the day, follow your personal preference. Climate is just something to consider when you pick your workout routine.

## Do You Prefer Exercising Alone or with People?

Some people prefer to get into their zone, be alone, put their headphones on, and just run. Others thrive on the motivation they get from a class environment with other students and a teacher to lead the way, such as with yoga, Pilates, or dance. Or possibly you prefer one-on-one attention from a personal trainer or a private yoga or Pilates instructor. What's your preference? There is no right or wrong answer. In fact, you don't even have to choose. You can always switch it up.

There is nothing better than yoga for a runner! Lots of runners are leery of doing yoga, because even though they are in shape, heart healthy, and lean, they might lack flexibility in their muscles from years of running. The strengthening and stretching of yoga are the perfect complements to running and any other sport. Knowing who you are and what environment

### TRENDING WORKOUTS

Capoeira: To strengthen, tone, and get lean

CrossFit: To strengthen, tone, and get lean

Kettlebells: To strengthen and tone

Pilates: To strengthen and tone

Spinning: To get lean

Tracy Anderson Method: To strengthen, tone, and get lean

Yoga: To strengthen and tone

suits you best will help you pick workouts that you will want to stick with.

## Do You Like to Play Sports?

If you grew up playing a sport, and it is something you love but haven't done in years, now is a perfect time to pick it up again. Tennis, golf, skiing, or even beach volleyball can be a great way to get in shape and socialize at the same time. You don't have to go to the gym for exercise to be considered a workout. We don't care if you never see the inside of a gym. Some people thrive when they compete, whether alone or on a team, so if sportsmanship and competition motivate you to get moving, great!

## What Is Your Budget?

Your budget will influence your choice of workout routine. Some things—like running and hiking outdoors—are free. Some activities—like skiing and golf, which require expensive equipment, plus lift tickets or course fees, etc.—can be pricey and not as accessible. Other activities—like yoga, spinning (studio cycling), or dance classes, or belonging to a gym—price out somewhere in the middle. Figure out what you can afford. We don't want money to be a deterrent to your getting your dream body. Maybe you set a compromise—scheduling one ski or golf trip a year and then finding another free or reasonably priced activity to do on a regular basis. Just think how in shape and ready you will be for that special trip when you have been exercising all year long!

## Do You Need Lessons?

Maybe this is your opportunity to learn something brand-new (surfing, anyone?) or to freshen up on a childhood activity you haven't practiced in years (horseback riding?). Committing to taking lessons is a great way to not only learn a new skill but also ensure you will stick with it. As with any type of learning, you need to

> ## HOW MUCH DOES IT COST?
>
> Gym membership: **$25 to $200 per month**
>
> Karate classes: **$50 to $100 per month (for three or more classes)**
>
> Personal trainer: **$50 to $100 and up per hour**
>
> Private yoga/Pilates instruction: **$75 to $100 and up per hour**
>
> Spinning class: **$15 to $25**
>
> Yoga/Pilates mat class: **$16 to $20**

practice (more than once a week!) to improve, so if you are taking a lesson once a week, make sure you have the ability and the access to practice at least two other times during the week. If you are taking tennis lessons, for example, you'll need access to courts and an opponent or a practice wall.

## Is This Something You Can Do at Least Three Times a Week?

Even if you don't need lessons, you need to be certain that whatever workout, exercise, or sport you choose, you will be able to practice it at least three times per

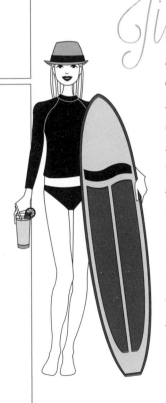

*Jill*

*I admit: I don't love working out. I dread it. However, I feel and look my best every time I do it, so I fight the urge to cancel on my trainer, bail on my spinning class, or not show up for my walk with friends in Central Park. I think the key is finding what you enjoy (as much as you can) and learning what works for your body. I have three main workouts. First, I train with kettlebells, a Russian technique where you swing a cast-iron weight (they come in different sizes) to combine cardiovascular exercise, strength training, and flexibility training. (My trainer Rich beats me up, and I love and hate him for it. He never lets me cancel. I once tried, but he banged on my door until I had to get up and work out. And you know what? It worked!) Second, I love spinning classes. I go to a place called SoulCycle. What I love about the sessions is they are only 45 minutes long and you fly through the entire workout! Third, I took up paddleboarding—essentially, standing on a surfboard and paddling around. It really works your core. I have reached (I'm proud to say) expert level and can paddle in all different types of environments. I was recently in Malibu in the Pacific Ocean, and as I was paddling, a dolphin swam right next to me. It was so incredible. (If you are on Facebook, check out my page. I have great pics!)*

week. If you can do it more frequently, all the better! And, yes, you can absolutely change it up. You don't have to do the same exact activity or play the same sport for all three workouts. You can go for a run, take a yoga class, and play a tennis match all in the same week. How much fun! Three times a week is the bare minimum; ideally, you will do something to move your body and feel great every day. Walking does count! Anytime you can walk instead of drive or take the stairs instead of the elevator, you should. When added together, even little changes to your activity level can count for a fourth workout in the week!

We've given you lots to think about and lots to look forward to. Now that you

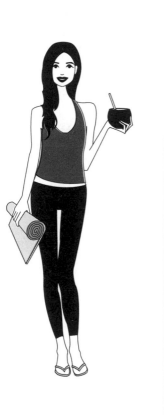

*Dana* *I like to think of myself as spontaneous, but when it comes to working out, I am a creature of habit. For the past 14 years, I have been practicing yoga as my main source of exercise. I love to hike, walk on the beach, or walk around the city, and depending on where I am, I will incorporate these in addition to my yoga. Prior to yoga, I was a spinning fanatic for about a year and a half. And before that, I ran on a treadmill at the gym (which I dreaded) or ran outside in the summer. I also consider myself a skier and a tennis player, but it has been an embarrassing 11 years since I have been on the slopes and about the same since I've been on a court. I know that yoga is something I love and will do for the rest of my life. It is such a part of my routine and of who I am that practice is automatic. So much so that I always go to the same yoga studio! I store my mat at my yoga studio, Virayoga in New York City, where I buy 20-class packs so I never have to think about attending or not attending, and I'm good to go.*

have your dream-body goal in sight and some idea about what workout routine would be fun and practical for you, get some rest. You are going to be active this weekend—perhaps more than you have been in a while.

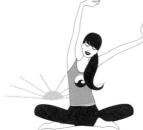

# SATURDAY MORNING

Have a nourishing breakfast, because now it's time to get down to business—real business, like signing up for dance classes (yes, *classes,* plural!), joining a gym, or hiring a trainer or pro. If you are thinking along the lines of exercising on your own outside, you will need to pick a route for your run, locate a hiking or biking trail, or find a pool in which to swim. (Search online for good running routes, public parks, hiking trails, or pools in your area; local and state government Web sites are a good source for this info.) If you choose to exercise with a partner or friend, obviously you will have to figure out together what you are both comfortable with and prepared to commit to.

**Pack your gym bag.** If you want variety, a visit to a gym may be your best bet. Most gyms nowadays have not only weights, treadmills, and bicycles but also a full schedule of different classes throughout the day (including yoga, Pilates, spinning, cross-training, and more), and some have extra amenities like rock-climbing walls and pools. A gym is also the perfect place to find and work out with a trainer, if that's what you want to do. Some gyms will include a couple of sessions with a trainer as an incentive to get you to join, which might be all

## WHICH CLASS TO CHOOSE?

Capoeira: **Strengthening, improves flexibility, cardiovascular, builds stamina**

Dance: **Aerobic, improves coordination and flexibility, fun**

Karate: **Strengthening; improves reflexes, coordination, and flexibility; confidence building; self-defense**

Pilates: **Strengthening, lengthening, increases flexibility, healing for injuries**

Yoga: **Strengthening, lengthening, increases flexibility, stress reducing, healing for injuries** you need to jump-start your workout routine. Training sessions will certainly alleviate any anxieties you might have about using unfamiliar equipment or what equipment settings are right for you.

Do a little online research to see what gyms are closest to your home or workplace, what the gyms offer, how much membership costs, and what's included in membership. (Tip: Ask the human resources department at your job whether your company gets a corporate discount at nearby gyms.) Maybe you have friends who can recommend a gym. If you can determine what establishment is right for you from this research, you're all set. If you'd like to see the facilities in person, plan to visit and take a tour today.

**Take a class.** If dance, yoga, Pilates, karate, or other classes are more up your alley, and you prefer to just pay for and attend those classes without joining a gym, then do some research to find a studio most suited for you. Good teachers and studios in these fields tend to get good word of mouth. With a bit of inquiry, you should be able to find one that is great and (hopefully) convenient. Some studios will let you take your first class for free. That way, you can try a class before you commit to 10 or 20 sessions or a monthlong pass. You are, however, committing to this practice as part of your workout makeover, so if you don't like your first teacher, keep trying until you find one or several who resonate with you. Pick a class to try this afternoon.

**Learn something new.** If golf, tennis, ice-skating, or any sport that requires lessons is going to be part of your regimen, finding a professional to teach you is your next step. Call your local public golf course, tennis court, or ice rink to get recommendations. You might not be able to book a lesson for today, but you can book one for this coming week! If you don't need coaching, and you just need to get off the couch, look online for info about hours and fees for public facilities in

## 10 SPORTS THAT REQUIRE LESSONS

1. Golf
2. Gymnastics
3. Horseback riding
4. Ice-skating
5. Paddleboarding
6. Rock climbing
7. Skiing
8. Surfing
9. Swimming
10. Tennis

*Jill* *When I am not on television, I am always in workout clothing. Always. My go-to outfit is Lululemon black pants, a cute T-shirt, and a hoodie sweatshirt. You do not need to spend a lot to look put-together in workout clothes. My favorite white T-shirts are from Target. (I also rock Converse sneakers from there.)*

*Dana* *I feel my best in general when I'm in a cute outfit. But when I'm exercising, I want to look cute and be comfortable. There's nothing more distracting than having to fidget and fix your outfit in the middle of your workout. When I am happy with my outfit, I feel good walking around the city or having lunch or running errands after my yoga class, even still dressed in my workout gear. Two of my fave yoga brands are Aziam and Beyond Yoga. And my new favorite shoes are the Vibram FiveFingers. They are fun and fashionable and give your feet a great stretch while you walk or run.*

your neighborhood. Either way, plan to play a little today, whether you hit golf balls at the driving range, hit tennis balls against a backboard, or take a few spins around the rink.

**Get outside.** If you prefer an outdoor workout—such as hiking, biking, running, or swimming—make a plan to do that today. There should be plenty of info online about public hiking trails, biking trails or bike lanes, and pools. If you want to run, local high schools often have tracks that provide a safe place to get in your workout; if you'd prefer to run on the streets, find a route that works for you and calculate how far you will go today.

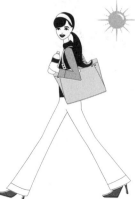

# ☀ SATURDAY AFTERNOON

We want you to be excited about this inspiring fitness adventure you are about to embark on, so in keeping with this weekend being all about you and achieving your goals, you deserve to treat yourself to a few motivational wardrobe items and gear, if necessary. This afternoon will be your first foray into your new regimen, and what better way to start than with a cute new outfit!

**Get in gear!** You have been diligent and done your research. You have picked what you want your workout to include. Congrats! Now it's time for a little shopping break. Let's hit the store. Most sporting goods stores sell merchandise for every activity imaginable, and, of course, there are specialty shops, too. Tons of places offer the perfect piece to fit within your budget. Check out Gap Body, Sports Authority, or even Target to find what you need.

If you have chosen one activity, purchase clothing and/or gear specific to that activity—a new pair of running shoes, a new tennis racquet, or a pair of yoga leggings, perhaps. If you plan to mix up your workouts, you can either buy clothing suitable for cross-training or splurge on something for each of your new activities. Although this is your preworkout reward, this isn't the time to hit the mall or your favorite boutique! That will be your reward for seeing the fruits of your labor after you have stuck to your routine for a bit. It only takes 21 days to make or break a habit, so let's see you make this one stick!

Now that you are properly geared up, let's get to it. There's no time like the present. Today is the

> ## 5 GREAT PREWORKOUT SNACKS
>
> 1. Almonds: 10–12 nuts
> 2. Oatmeal: 1 cup
> 3. Fruit: Banana, apple, peach
> 4. Trail mix: ½ cup with nuts, seeds, dried fruit
> 5. Yogurt: 8 ounces low-fat plain flavor

*Jill* If I haven't stressed this enough, I hate working out!
Again, I know I must do it, and I know each and every
day is better when I do. I have one rule, though, and this
pertains to all of my workouts: They must be done in
the morning. So if I am going to the Today show at 6:30 a.m.
for a 9:00 a.m. segment, I will get up at 5:00 to train. If I
don't do it in the morning, first thing, it ain't happening!
My only request: a cup of coffee. My trainer Rich stops
and gets coffee for us. Everyone should have a motivator.
Find a loved one who will hook you up with whatever
gets you going!

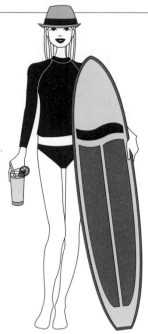

*Dana* I have worked out at every time of day, and my
workouts are definitely better in the evening—I am more limber,
I have less on my mind, and the exercise eases me right into
a great night's sleep. However, I know myself, and unless I am
going straight from the office to a yoga class, exercise doesn't
happen unless I go in the morning. So on the weekends
(and because I work from home), I work out in the morning.
Exercising is a priority, and doing it first thing enables
me to check it off my to-do list. Believe me, I still get the same
results and same great feeling from a morning class! I love
starting my day this way.

beginning of your new regimen and your new life. Grab a light bite or a smoothie to sustain you if you are hungry, and get ready to hit the gym, the trail, the pool, the court, the course, your very first yoga class, or whatever it is that you have chosen.

You will be amazed at how much more effort it takes to get somewhere the first time than it takes every time after that (which is why you will be coming back tomorrow, too!). Truly, we understand. New environments can be uncomfortable or intimidating—all the people around you seem to know what they are doing and where they are going. But remember: Everyone else had a first day once, too. And guess what? No one is really looking at you like you don't belong—it just seems like they are. In reality, everyone is there for the same reason: to get their workout on. To calm your first-day jitters, you might want to bring a friend along, someone to hold your hand (a trainer can soften the experience, too). But if you go solo, that's absolutely fine. We are here, rooting for you, telling you that you *can* do this, and you know you can, too. You have done the research, you are on time, and you look fabulous in the outfit you just bought. Now all you need to do is focus, participate, and have *fun*!

Finished with your first session? Be proud of yourself. We are proud of you. What an amazing first day. You got in the game and got started. You should feel energized yet relaxed and full of endorphins. You might feel a little sore tomorrow (or maybe a lot!), depending on what kind of shape you are in and how much you exerted yourself, but muscle fatigue is one of the greatest sensations. It reminds you that you did something good for yourself; your body is letting you know that you got results.

> ## 5 BEST POSTWORKOUT MEALS AND SNACKS
>
> 1. Protein shake: Protein powder with either milk or dairy substitute and fruit
> 2. Piece of grilled fish and sautéed spinach
> 3. Beans and rice and steamed broccoli
> 4. Salad with grilled chicken
> 5. Egg omelette with veggies

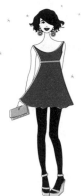

## SATURDAY NIGHT

Now it's time to pamper yourself. This weekend is for you, so as hard as you've been working, we want you to relax and enjoy this workout makeover, too. Your muscles will appreciate a soak in a nice hot bath, and you can use Epsom salts to soothe them if they are sore. Take the time to luxuriate and let everything go. Shut your eyes and breathe deeply. When you're done, use moisturizer or body oil and massage your muscles a bit. (If you have a partner, and you can convince him to massage your muscles for you, even better!) You'll be happy you did your workout this morning.

After the bath (or before, if you're starving), get cozy and have a delicious, healthy, and nutritious dinner. Remember that a hard workout is not license to eat whatever you want! When you are feeling good about your body, which you should be after a great workout, you'll tend to want to eat better, too. The more good things you do for yourself, the more you will want to do. It's the opposite of a vicious cycle, so embrace it!

Another super benefit of working out is a restful night's sleep. Your body will be ready to drift off into a deep slumber, so keep tonight mellow and take advantage of the opportunity to catch up on some z's.

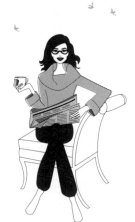

## SUNDAY

How do you feel this morning? You might be a little sore, but we bet it's a good sore, right? This is a reminder that you did something new, something incredible, and something ultimately rewarding for yourself. The sensation might be a little unfamiliar or uncomfortable, but we have the perfect remedy.

**Do it again!** Yes, we want you to exercise again today. And, no, this does not mean another stint on the rock-

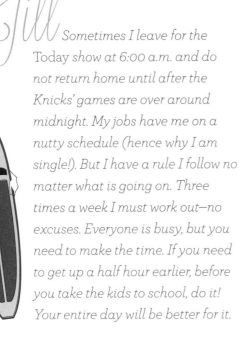

*Jill* Sometimes I leave for the
*Today* show at 6:00 a.m. and do
not return home until after the
Knicks' games are over around
midnight. My jobs have me on a
nutty schedule (hence why I am
single!). But I have a rule I follow no
matter what is going on. Three
times a week I must work out—no
excuses. Everyone is busy, but you
need to make the time. If you need
to get up a half hour earlier, before
you take the kids to school, do it!
Your entire day will be better for it.

*Dana* I practice
yoga three or four times per week.
Generally, I go to the same
classes, but sometimes my work
or personal schedule requires
that I switch it around, so not
every week looks exactly the
same. On days that I can't get to
the yoga studio, or I choose to do
something else, I make sure I get
in a long walk. And whenever I
have the choice, I always opt for
taking the stairs instead of an
escalator or elevator!

climbing wall, a grueling match of tennis, or an energetic dance class, but we do want you to move your body today. This could mean a long walk, a light swim, or a gentle yoga class—anything that will get your body moving to keep you in the habit of doing something physical.

We know it might not be realistic to fit in a workout every single day, but the more often you exercise, the more often you will want to do it. The sooner and faster you can make exercise a habit, the better. It's addicting, really, in the very best way.

You have dedicated this weekend to getting your fitness regimen in gear so that you can get your body in the best shape possible. While you have this rare opportunity, this precious weekend, take advantage and get in a second workout.

There is nothing better than another yoga class to alleviate some of the soreness from yesterday's yoga class. Stretching and moving is what you need to do to get your muscles to relax and let go. The soreness is mostly just the muscles tightening up while you were sleeping in reaction to their use yesterday.

This morning, pick a fitness activity that you would like to do today. You can decide whether you want to get up and go right away or whether you'd like to relax a bit and head out in the afternoon. Everyone has a different preference for what time they feel best working out. Some people like to get up and immediately work out, because they know themselves: They know if exercise doesn't happen in the morning, it's not going to happen at all. If this describes you, don't fight your personality—work with it. Get up and just go before you have time to think about it. If you prefer an afternoon or evening workout and you know you will actually do it, that's great, too. If you are participating with other people in perhaps a round of golf or a tennis game, sometimes the commitment of the date is enough that you will go regardless of the time of day. Group activities are especially nice on the weekend because they are social, too.

Whatever activity you select is fine with us, as long as you choose to do something. You are going to feel amazing once you start to move, but you won't believe us until you do it!

**Plan ahead to stay active.** There is one more thing you must do today. Once

## 6 PERKS OF A MORNING WORKOUT

1. You get it done and checked off your list first thing.

2. You don't have time to talk yourself out of going.

3. You won't miss the workout if you have to work late.

4. You get your metabolism going and your mind and body loosened up and ready for the day.

5. You are free to make social plans in the evening.

6. You are able to fall asleep at night without being amped up from an evening workout.

## 5 PERKS OF AN EVENING WORKOUT

1. You don't have to get up extra early if you are not a morning person.

2. Your body is already warmed up from the day and not stiff from sleeping, so your body will be more open and flexible in the evening.

3. You can get in a longer workout if you are not rushed to get to work or start your day.

4. You've already eaten throughout the day, so you will be less hungry after your workout.

5. Exercise is a great way to clear your mind after a busy day to make for a better night's sleep.

you've sorted out an activity and a time for your exercise, set aside time to map out your fitness regimen. To stick to your routine, you need to schedule your workouts into your busy week. To ensure that they happen, enter them in your calendar.

Take out your date book or smartphone or whatever tool you use to keep appointments, and look at your schedule. Find three time slots per week to fit in a workout. If you want to and can fit in more slots, fantastic. If not, let's just start with the three. You can break this down however you like. Maybe you want to do something twice during the workweek and once over the weekend. It's better to spread out the sessions so that you don't have three days of exercise in a row followed by four off. For example, maybe you choose Monday, Wednesday, and Saturday. Or you prefer Tuesday, Thursday, and Sunday. If you want your weekends free, then maybe you flag Monday, Wednesday, and Friday. If you have the time to fit in three workouts during the week, then may we be so bold as to suggest that over the weekend you sneak in a fourth just by being social and going for a hike or playing tennis with your partner or friends!

The day and time can fluctuate every week. We understand that things come up, and not every week contains exactly the same amount of work, appointments, commitments, etc. But once you start blocking out time for exercise in your schedule, just as you do for any other weekly appointment, it will become habit.

Take the time today to figure out what is realistic for you. If you have an office job, decide whether you are going to get up earlier two or three times per week and hit the gym, studio, court, track, what have you, before work, or if you would rather pack your workout gear and go straight after work. Again, this is a totally personal preference based on your time availability and whether you are a morning person or a night person. There is no right or wrong here, as long as you show up.

**Feel free to switch it up.** The first week, try exercising before work. If that doesn't suit you, the following week try going after work. Some people even sneak their workout into their lunch hour.

Other factors beyond time of day can influence your exercise period. Perhaps you like one of the morning classes better, or your trainer is only available in the evening. Maybe you prefer to change up your workout in the summer versus the winter—by taking advantage of longer, warmer days and being outside. Whatever you decide to do this first week, it is not set in stone; you can make changes next week. What it does mean is that you must take time every Sunday to plan and schedule your workout for the week. Once you figure out what's best for you—time of day, favorite teachers, workout preferences—workouts will become second nature. The first 3 weeks are crucial in forming the habit of just getting yourself exercising.

Now that you have planned (or completed) your workout for today, and have scheduled your fitness regimen for the week, you should feel motivated and pretty proud. We are proud of you! Starting a workout routine is no small feat, but you have it under control. There is nothing better than when you start feeling—and seeing—results! Truly, once you get on the fitness bandwagon, you won't want to get off. Moving your body feels so great that you might even forget why you got started in the first place!

Take this day to eat healthy—three core meals and some good-for-you snacks (refer to Chapter 1 for ideas). No indulging or overeating just because you completed two great workouts this weekend. Your dream body will develop only if you take care of your current body by moving it, nourishing it, and resting it. There is no other way.

Be nice to yourself and your body, and indulge in another nice hot bath or get a massage after your workout. You deserve it! Relax after this active and productive weekend makeover and get ready for an amazing week ahead.

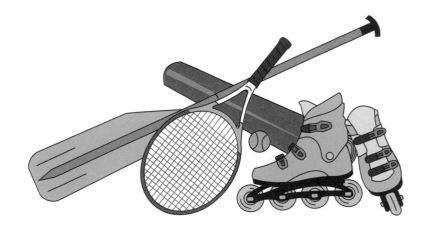

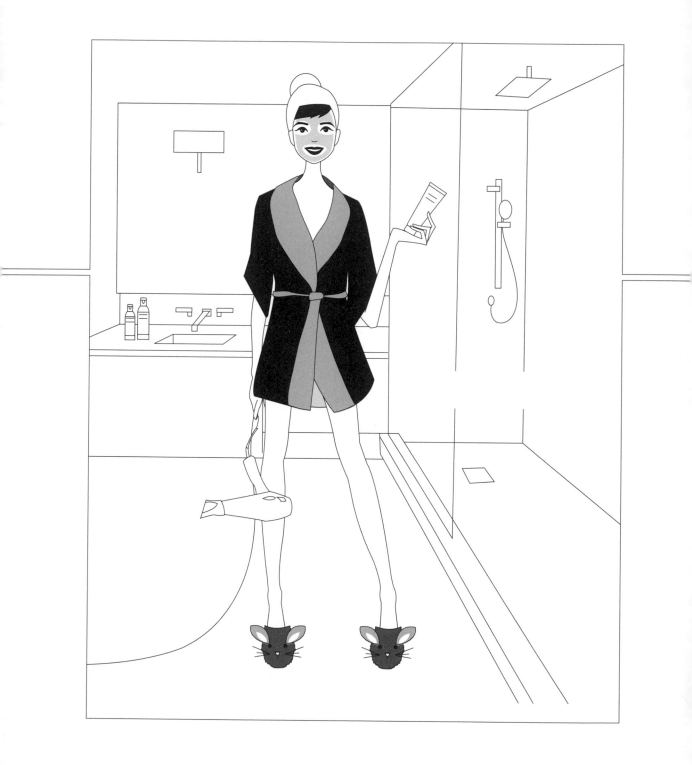

# Chapter Three
# Beauty Makeover

Are you in a beauty rut? Do you wish you knew how to apply your makeup like the celebrities? Do you wish you had the time to apply makeup, period? Have you let your skin care routine slide? Or rather, is your answer, "*What* skin care routine?" Beauty—and appearance—is another area that we tend to neglect in our busy lives. While addressing beauty might not seem as crucial as getting your diet or workout on track, putting a fresh face forward is just as important to your self-esteem. One study by the University of California, Berkeley, found that people could accurately judge another person's personality traits based on full-body photographs alone. The upshot: Your clothing style, facial expressions, and posture say a lot about your personality.

Truly, this is an area that, with a few easy lessons and a little bit of positive habit forming, can be changed almost overnight—well, in a weekend anyway! Are you ready to give yourself this weekend to beautify and recharge? You deserve it! Of course, there's a desire to be your most beautiful self for the current or future man in your life, but more important, you should want to look glowing and gorgeous for yourself!

This weekend, we are going to walk you through implementing a skin care routine that you can maintain every day. You'll find a few go-to makeup looks that will have you radiant, ready, and out the door in no time.

## ☾ FRIDAY NIGHT

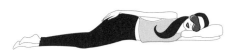

We know it's there: in your medicine cabinet, on your vanity, or in your makeup case. Yes, we are talking about makeup or moisturizer from 1991. We are all guilty of hoarding old beauty products. Most people have a ton of products and don't even know what half of them are for—and they certainly don't use them! Instead of trying to decipher your supplies, the first step is to do a massive cleanout (unless you bought something recently and actually use it) and start fresh, clean, and new. By the end of this weekend makeover, you'll be surprised at how little you actually do need.

First things first. This evening begins a weekend that is all about you—a mini-break to celebrate the fabulous you who's waiting to emerge. It will be a weekend to transform but also to relax and enjoy. Would you rather clean out and then relax over a nice, healthy dinner and a glass of wine, or would you rather relax first and then get to work? Totally up to you—but make it a fun Friday night, even though you're getting down to business!

**Decide what to let go.** Tonight, you have an "evening in" to attack the bathroom, your purse, your travel kit, and anywhere else a stash of makeup or skin care products lurks. Even though makeup is packaged and stored in plastic and looks like it lasts for years, here's the reality: Makeup has an expiration date. This is especially true for liquids, such as mascara and lip gloss, which are susceptible to bacteria growth. We know it's hard to toss out a perfectly pretty gloss, but it's not worth risking infection. And the great thing about makeup is it's not like an expensive dress—for under $10 you can get something new!

Discard mascara after 3 months—but if your mascara starts to dry up *before* 90 days, throw it away. Mascara has the shortest life span of all makeup because the risk of transferring bacteria from your eye to the mascara tube is so high. Adding water or saliva only increases your chances of getting an eye infection.

Eyeliner pencils can be kept for up to 3 years, but sharpen the tip before each application to make sure it's clean. Lipstick and lip gloss are good for up to 1 year. Sharpen your lip pencil just as with your eye pencil. If you keep your applicators, then liquid eye shadows should last you a year, while powder shadows can keep for up to 2 years. If you've had an eye infection in the past, toss all of your eye makeup—using it again will cause another infection. Get rid of your cream blushes after a year, and all powders after 2 years.

> ## TOP 10 MAKEUP PRODUCTS' SHELF LIFE
>
> 1. Cleanser: **6–12 months**
> 2. Concealer: **Up to 1 year**
> 3. Eyeliner pencil: **3 years with regular sharpening**
> 4. Eye shadow: **2 years (powder), 1 year (liquid)**
> 5. Foundation: **6–12 months**
> 6. Lip gloss/lipstick: **1 year**
> 7. Lip liner pencil: **3 years with regular sharpening**
> 8. Mascara: **3 months**
> 9. Moisterizer: **6 months**
> 10. Powder/blush: **Up to 2 years**

Because many makeup and beauty products can be inexpensive impulse buys, it's easy to be swayed by advertising, trends, and pretty packaging and end up buying a ton of stuff you don't need and never use. Let's remedy that right now. Clear off a table or make a pile on the floor (wherever you have the most room) and put all of your makeup products there. Amazing how much is there when you see it together!

Start with one category at a time. We'll work with skin care first. We're guessing you have a ton of different cleansers, creams, toners, masks, and exfoliants. You are correct that these products are useful, and tomorrow you'll get a set of these that work together and are appropriate for your skin type, but right now we want you to ask yourself the following about each item:

1. How old is it?
2. Do you like the product's texture and scent?
3. Does it match other products by the same brand?
4. Is it the right product for your skin type?
5. Do you use it at least once per week?

If you don't remember when you bought it, toss it. If you don't like the texture or the scent, toss it. If you have a bunch of different products that are not part of a set or within the same brand, toss 'em. If you didn't take into account, or have never paid attention to, your skin type and are not sure these products are appropriate for you, yes, toss 'em! And if you don't use it at least once a week, well . . .

Now let's look at your makeup. When was the last time you dumped out your makeup bag? We can just imagine what you have stashed in there! We're guessing you have any or all of these: eyeliners, eye shadows, mascaras, brow gels, brow pencils, blushes, foundations, powders, lip liners, lipsticks, lip glosses, and concealers, not to mention all the tools (blush brushes, eye shadow brushes, eyelash curlers, lip brushes, and tweezers). We know that winnowing through these products can be overwhelming, so where to begin? Let's take a look at each item:

1. How old is it?
2. When was the last time you used it?
3. Did you buy the color because it was trendy?
4. Do you have duplicates of the same product?

If it is liquid that uses an applicator that has touched your lips or eyes and is older than 3 months, toss it. If it is a pencil or a powder and is still usable, be

*Jill* I know this is a generalization, but most men (and women) prefer a woman with less makeup, or at least one who looks like she is wearing little makeup! I am a big believer in the rule that less is more. I grew up with terrible skin. (The kids called me Pizza Face. I won't name names, but Jeffery is the boy who used to tease me the most. Not that I hold grudges!) My main concern is that my skin appears clear and glowing. I do not spend a ton of money on department store lines or fancy products. My dermatologist gave me a regimen I follow every day. I wash my face with a machine called Clarisonic twice a day. (You can get it at Sephora.) It is a little pricey, but it gets my skin totally clean. Five days a week I have TV makeup on, so it takes a small army (or small machine!) to remove it all. When I am not working, my daytime look is simple: concealer under my eyes, bronzer, and a nude lip gloss.

*Dana* I try to keep my beauty routine simple and easy. I don't wear a lot of makeup. In fact, I don't wear any, except if I'm going out at night, attending an event, or doing something where I will be photographed or on TV. When I wear makeup, my basics are eye shadow, brow gel, mascara, eyeliner, and lip balm—I don't even go full-on with the lipstick or gloss! However, I do keep my skin looking great. I never go to sleep with makeup on. Studies have shown that not only does sleeping with makeup cause acne, but also mascara flakes may end up in your eye, causing itchiness, bloodshot eyes, infections, or eye scratches. I wash and moisturize every day. I exfoliate several times a week, use toner when I need a little something extra, and apply a face mask when I want to treat myself. I am also a big fan of the sun, so I try to maintain a bit of a tan to keep my skin looking even and healthy.

## 6 BASIC SKIN TYPES

1. Dry
2. Oily
3. Problem
4. Sensitive
5. Aging or damaged
6. Normal

honest—when was the last time you used it? If you don't remember, toss it. Take stock of all the different colors of eye shadows, lipsticks, eyeliners, etc., that you have. Do you really wear the coral lipstick or the turquoise eye shadow, or did it just look pretty on a swimsuit model in a magazine last summer? Be honest! Sometimes the idea of something is better than the reality. If you bought it but never use it, toss it.

Do you have six brown eyeliners, 20 eye shadow palettes, and four bottles of foundation in various shades? We thought so. Guess what? You don't need them all. It's time to pare down, to trim the excess, and to get into a functioning beauty routine. Do you need one set of makeup for at home and another to tote around in your purse? If so, then you can keep duplicate items in both places. We want to make sure you are sorted with the right products, so starting from scratch, or as close to it as possible, is the best way to go.

As for brushes, curlers, and tweezers, these are good to have on hand. They get damaged, though, so make sure yours are in working order. If bristles are bent or missing, it's time to replace the brushes. If the curler isn't working well, try cleaning it with a little warm water and makeup remover, if necessary, carefully removing all makeup residue. Don't forget to replace the curler's rubber insert every 3 months, as that does wear and dry out. Tweezers, if dropped, can get bent, which makes them less effective. These also need to be cleaned to make sure they are precise. Some companies, like Tweezerman, offer free lifetime sharpening.

It may seem painful to throw away so much makeup, but trust us—a major purge is a necessary step toward a streamlined, easy-to-manage beauty routine. You will be so happy when you go into the bathroom or peek into your makeup bag and see only the products you need for a fresh and glowing face!

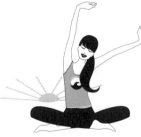

# SATURDAY MORNING

Now that you've purged your bathroom and makeup bag of unnecessary products, you'll want to restock with the right skin care products that are geared toward your exact skin care needs. How do you know what's right?

Take a good look at your skin this morning as soon as you wake up. Is it dry and flaky, or is it a bit oily? Do you have problems with acne, or are you prone to breakouts? Have you ever had an allergic reaction to any skin product? Is your skin damaged from sun or aging? Or would you say your skin is pretty much problem free and you haven't noticed any of the above?

Before you go shopping for beauty supplies, take this morning to think about your lifestyle, your personality, your age, and your coloring.

**Lifestyle.** How do you spend your days and your nights? Do you work at an office or from home? Do you spend your days running from activity to activity with your kids? Do you attend a lot of business functions or social functions or spend fun evenings out on the town? All of these factors will determine the kinds of makeup looks you might want to try. Obviously, heavier, dramatic looks are more appropriate at night. You never want to overdo it at the office or on the soccer field. And even at night, less is always more. The heavy-handed '80s look is definitely out!

**Personality.** Your face (and, of course, your makeup) is the first thing people see when they meet you, so you want to be comfortable and give off an impression that is genuinely you. A lot can be said by the amount and type of makeup you wear. If you are creative, maybe you wear makeup that makes an edgy or interesting statement. If you are conservative, your makeup should be, too. If you are loud and outgoing, maybe you want to experiment with brighter or more daring makeup. Regardless, makeup is supposed to enhance your look, not hide it or make you look like you are in costume. When in doubt, going for a natural look that gives you an extra lift is always your best bet.

**Age.** A big misconception is that the older you get, the heavier the makeup you need. This is absolutely *not* the case. In fact, the heavier your makeup, the older you will appear. Another big no-no is trying too hard to look younger by incorporating all the latest makeup trends and colors. Figure out what makeup colors look best on you and learn how to apply them. That is the surest way to put your best face forward. If bright red lipstick is a trend, there is no harm in experimenting, but be true to yourself when you look in the mirror. Is that red really you? If so, go for it. If not, that's fine, too.

**Coloring.** Take into consideration your skin tone and your hair color when choosing makeup looks. For the most part, natural colors—anything in the brown family—will look good on everyone. If you are going to experiment with shadow colors or lip colors, take the following into account. If you are blonde, redheaded, or gray with fair or pale skin, cooler colors will be flattering—greens, blues, purples, and grays on the eyes and lip color with blue (or cool) undertones. If you are a brunette with medium, dark, or olive skin, warmer colors will be most flattering—browns, golds, pinks, and peaches on the eyes and lip color with warm undertones.

**Get inspired.** Feel free to browse fashion and beauty magazines to find looks that you want to try. Tear out your favorite pages to bring to the store and keep yourself on track so you don't buy too much new makeup. You'd be surprised how many different looks you can achieve with one product. You can go from day to night, or natural to dramatic, by applying the makeup a bit more heavily. A smoky eye requires the same eye makeup as an everyday look. It's just how heavily and where on the eye you apply it. Aside from maybe a few color choices in eye shadow or lip color, the rest of your makeup will be composed of the basics.

Most beauty magazines (and the beauty section of fashion magazines) will show you how to re-create the look in the picture, so you will have instructions on exactly how to apply the makeup this evening when you start to experiment. If you prefer that someone teach you how, many department stores and beauty stores (like Sephora) offer personal consultations. Most times these are free, but the sales reps will often suggest you buy their makeup. Don't feel pressured to make a big purchase just because they've given you a makeover! Simply thank them for their help and decide for yourself what you need or want.

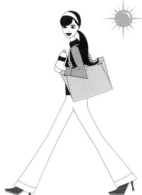

# SATURDAY AFTERNOON

It's up to you where to shop for new beauty supplies. Truthfully, the makeup will look the same on your face whether you buy it at a department store, the drugstore, or a beauty supply store. These days, many drugstores have an extensive beauty section, where you can pretty much find everything you need at affordable prices.

The price point is obviously higher at department stores, but you will get the aid of a full-service professional sales staff and on-site makeup artists. And don't forget—this is your weekend to dedicate to improving the way you look and feel. Why shouldn't you hop on the chair and have your makeup done? It doesn't matter if you have plans later or are just planning to relax at home. Today is your day. Take the time, have a seat, and get a makeover—you'll feel fabulous!

**Make a list.** If you're a total minimalist and only wear moisturizer and a little concealer, then a quick trip to the drugstore or beauty supply store should do the trick. But most of us need a few additional products. It's helpful to have a list handy so you're not tempted to fill up your bathroom with more of the same stuff you just got rid of!

## SKIN CARE BASICS

1. Facial cleanser

2. Toner

3. Facial moisturizer (If you want one with SPF for during the day, then you will need that plus a night cream.)

4. Exfoliating face scrub

5. Face mask

Ideally, purchase all of these products from the same brand, as they are made with ingredients that work together as a system to achieve the best results. Also, keep in mind what you discovered this morning regarding your skin type. It's important that your products are healing and soothing, so you want to get ones geared to your particular skin type.

## MAKEUP BASICS

1. Eyeliner or eye pencil
2. Mascara
3. Eye shadow palette or separates (You will need four complementary shades to create any look. This is easy, as they usually come in sets of four.)
4. Blush or bronzer
5. Lipstick or lip gloss
6. Brow gel
7. Concealer
8. Translucent powder

## ADD-ONS

1. Foundation
2. Lip pencil
3. Brow pencil

The first eight products—the makeup basics—are the bare-bone necessities to put together a basic "look." If you are simply wanting a bit of enhancement, you might need just a little blush, mascara, and lip gloss. If you want to take your look a step further, you can add the lip and brow pencils for more definition. Foundation is a personal preference. Some women won't leave the house without it, and some prefer to keep their skin bare. And if you found a look that you want to try this weekend and it requires certain colors—red lipstick, for example, or purple eye shadow—be sure you pick up these products, too. (If you're experimenting, you might want to purchase a less-expensive drugstore brand until you commit to a look that you will proudly wear.)

The basics and add-ons don't have to be the same brand, but organizationally and aesthetically, it is nice to have everything uniform. It also makes shopping easier and faster when you can stick to one section of the store. People gravitate toward certain brands according to personal preferences—pretty packaging, the ad campaign, or a recommendation from a friend, salesperson, or makeup artist. Whatever brand, or brands, you choose is fine as long as it makes you happy.

## MAKEUP TOOLS

You'll also want to have the following tools on hand:

1. Blush brush (can be used for blush, powder, and bronzer)
2. Eye shadow brush (better than the spongy small thingies that come in the eye shadow case, and you can clean it, too!)
3. Makeup pencil sharpener (to keep your eye, lip, and brow pencils sharp, clean, and easy to apply)
4. Eyelash curler
5. Eyebrow tweezers
6. Makeup remover (any body oil will serve the same purpose)
7. Q-tips (to help apply or remove makeup)
8. Cotton balls (to help remove makeup)

These tools will be useful in maintaining your beauty routine. And

## 5 PROS AND CONS OF ORGANIC MAKEUP

1. Organic makeup uses natural ingredients that are healthier for you, compared with traditional makeup that uses synthetic chemicals that can be damaging or toxic.

2. Because organic makeup uses only natural dyes, the color choices are more limited.

3. The coverage of organic makeup is lighter, so it masks imperfections; traditional makeup is heavier and can get into lines and wrinkles, causing them to stand out more.

4. Traditional makeup can be easier to apply because of its smoother texture.

5. Organic makeup is generally hypoallergenic and free from dyes and fragrances that can irritate sensitive skin.

while you're at the store and in fresh-start mode, go ahead and splurge a little—get yourself some new razors, body oil or moisturizer, and a new toothbrush, too!

**Consider organic products.** If you are concerned about the ingredients used in your makeup and skin care products, as well as about issues of packaging, environmental safety, and animal testing, you may want to shop at a health foods market such as Whole Foods. But read labels carefully: The Environmental Working Group says that even plant-based ingredients can be harmful and should meet the same safety standard as those derived from petroleum, mines, or animals. It's hard to tell which ingredients are truly organic or natural, because truth-in-marketing rules for food don't apply in the cosmetics world. An exception are products with the USDA organic seal, which contain ingredients from plants grown without artificial pesticides and fertilizers.

When you get home, unpack and set up all of your new products in your beautifully empty bathroom or on your cleaned-off vanity. Make some fabulous plans for tonight—either a date with your man or a fun night out with the girls. This is going to be your first outing with your new look!

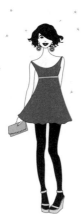

# SATURDAY NIGHT

Whether or not you've made fun plans for this evening, treat yourself to a nice hot bath or decadently long shower. Make sure your face is completely cleaned off (using your new cleanser and moisturizer) if you wore any makeup earlier. Put on your robe and get ready to play!

The goal here is to find an evening/night-out makeup look that works for your lifestyle, personality, age, and coloring and that you can easily apply. We know it's not every day, or every weekend even, that you will have the time to spend getting ready to go out. Lots of times, you are juggling the kids while dressing and barely make it out the door on time. But not tonight. Tonight, you are going to invest the time so that, in the future, applying cosmetics will be a no-brainer.

If you had your makeup done by a pro earlier, he or she should have walked

# 10 TIPS TO ENHANCE NATURAL BEAUTY

1. Keep your face clean, exfoliated, and moisturized for a young fresh look.
2. Keep brows groomed.
3. Use a powdered blush/bronzer for an allover glow.
4. Use a little clear lip balm or gloss to polish your pucker.
5. Use mascara to enhance your natural lashes without looking overdone.
6. Eat healthy.
7. Stay hydrated by drinking plenty of water.
8. Exercise regularly to keep the blood flowing and the muscles in your face relaxed.
9. Get at least 8 hours of sleep per night.
10. Dab a little tea tree oil on blemishes to make them disappear quickly.

you through the steps to apply everything. If not, get out your magazine instructions and follow along. You don't have to wear your makeup the same way every time, but learning how to apply it and finding a go-to look will make your life easier and getting ready that much quicker. Once applying your makeup is part of your routine, you shouldn't need much longer than 10 minutes for your daytime look and no more than 20 for an evening look.

**Find your personal makeup style.** Just as in fashion, makeup has trends, too. Smoky eyes, red lips, and thicker or thinner brows all come in and out of vogue. Trendy looks are definitely fun to experiment with, but as with clothing, it is always better to have your own personal style, one that will never go out of fashion, than it is to follow every trend that comes along. So let's focus on developing your personal makeup style.

By now you should have a brand-new makeup palette composed of colors and tones that work for your skin coloring. General rule: If you are going to go darker or heavy-handed on the lip—a true red lip, for example—go lighter and more

## Jill

*When my mother was growing up, she overdid it with her eyebrows. After too many years of plucking them too thin, she now has to draw them on! (Sorry to throw you under the bus, Mom, but hopefully your story will help others.) Eyebrows shape your face and make a difference in your overall look. I consulted an aesthetician I trust, and she shaped them for me. I then had my brows permanently shaped with electrolysis. This treatment removes hair (pretty much forever). I am happy I did it—it's one less thing to have to worry about.*

## Dana

*I am obsessed with eyebrows. For whatever reason (probably because it was trendy), I started tweezing my eyebrows to be thinner years ago. I used to do it myself, and then when I was living in LA, I went to Jacqui, the eyebrow girl. She was a real artist (painter) and a makeup artist, but she mainly did eyebrows; she was great. I have since maintained them on my own, but now that the trend has been for thicker, more natural brows, I have been letting them grow back in. It is a long process, and they are not what they were when I look back at pictures from years ago. Word to the wise—no matter what the trend, don't overpluck!*

natural on the eye area. Vice versa if you are doing a smoky or heavier eye look— go natural on the lips and cheeks. You want to make one feature the focal point— sort of like how you accessorize with jewelry!

Keep in mind the four things we asked you to consider before you went shopping—lifestyle, personality, age, and coloring. Red lips are a big statement, as are smoky eyes, so if you are trying any makeup trend that makes a bold statement, be sure that you're comfortable before you walk out of the house. Otherwise, a basic makeup look that shows off your best face is all you need. Remember, you're already awesome! Makeup is just a tool to inject an extra kick of confidence before you greet the world.

**Start with your brows.** Before you put on makeup, get out your tweezers and take a look at your brows. Make sure you have enough light near the mirror so you can see what's going on. (If you don't have good lighting or a window with natural light in your bathroom, you might invest in a portable makeup mirror

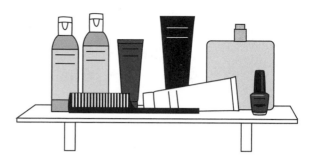

with built-in lighting so you can really see what you are doing.) Let us first mention that trends in brow thickness change with the times, but the best thing you can do for yourself in this department is to keep your natural brows and just clean up between them (between your eyes) and remove any strays below your brow bone.

The trick is this: Looking in a mirror, hold a pencil straight up and down alongside your nose and tweeze anything on the inside of that line (closest to your nose). Then hold the pencil straight up and down over the very center (pupil) of your eye looking straight ahead: Anything to the outside (away from your nose) that is underneath the natural brow line can be plucked.

You never want to end up with gaps in the brow line or with brows that are too thin—even when thinner brows are "in." It is difficult to grow them back, and they don't always come back in fully. Your brows frame your face, so you don't want to mess with this! If you are nervous, have your brows expertly shaped by a professional first. Then you can maintain them yourself using the pro's work as a guide. Be sure to get a referral or see examples of someone's work before you entrust yourself to her or him so you aren't unpleasantly surprised by the results.

**Finish off your look.** Once you have a clean face and perfect brows, continue on to concealer. Cover any blemishes or dark circles under the eyes. If you are using foundation, that comes next. If not, move on to the eyes. Shadow first—the medium color goes on your eyelid, the darkest color in the lid crease, and the lightest color goes on the brow bone, just under your eyebrow. Next, apply eyeliner on the outside of the top lid, just along the lash line. If you want a heavier look, apply liner underneath your bottom lashes, too. Then curl your top lashes

*Jill* *I think you have more choices when you limit your choices. What I mean is that your makeup bag—whether it's at home or on the go—shouldn't be a disaster. You should not have 10 mascaras, 400 lip glosses, and 60 blushes. Pick the colors that you actually use and that look best on your skin tone, and get rid of the rest. Everything should be neat and in order when you are getting ready (day or night). No need for extra clutter. Ever.*

*Dana* *As I mentioned, I don't wear much in the way of makeup during the day, but there are two must-haves in my makeup arsenal that I don't leave the house without. The first is Brow Set, a clear brow grooming gel from MAC Cosmetics. The second is Karite Lips, a shea butter-based, vanilla-scented all-natural lip balm from Mode de Vie.*

and apply mascara—again to just the top lashes or to both, if you want a more dramatic look. Next, groom your brows with either clear brow gel or the color you bought that matches your brows. Add a little blush along the cheekbones, then some translucent powder all over your face to set your look. Finally, put on some lipstick or gloss, and for a more dramatic look, you can add some lip liner. Voilà!

**Feel free to experiment.** We walked you through a complete makeup look using all your supplies, but there is no right or wrong here. Try a look using eyeliner and no shadow, or shadow and no liner. Try lining either the top or the bottom of the eye, or line both. Try a darker eye and a lighter lip, and vice versa. Find what works for you. The products you will want to use regardless of the other style choices are your mascara, blush, brow gel, and some sort of lip enhancer—even if it's just a clear gloss.

The details of your evening plans, and the people you will be with, will determine how heavy-handed and daring you will be on any given night. (With your makeup look, of course!) Play around a bit and see what you like. Your eyes and lips will be the features that have the most play as far as switching up the look. (You have a brand-new jar of eye-makeup remover at the ready!) Find a look that's perfect for a date night of dinner and a movie, and another that would be a bit more dramatic for attending a wedding or other formal affair. Once you get comfortably in the groove applying your makeup, little nuances will be a piece of cake and can change with your mood or your plans.

**Don't forget to take it all off.** Whether you had a blast out with friends tonight or simply enjoyed a quiet evening at home, it's time for your beauty sleep. But not so fast! Your skin won't look so beautiful in the morning if you go to sleep wearing a full face of makeup, and we wouldn't want to see your pillowcase in the morning, either!

We know you are tired, but take the time to start your skin care regimen. That's what this weekend is for. No time like the present for forming a new habit.

First, take off your eye makeup with the remover or a little body oil and a cotton ball. This will make for much less mess when you wash your face. Then wash your face thoroughly with your new cleanser. Grab another cotton ball and apply the toner on your face, making sure to get all around the sides—by your ears, forehead, and your neck. The toner removes any makeup residue and gives your face a fresh, tingly feeling. Next, moisturize. (Most makeup is made using synthetic chemicals, dyes, and fragrances that can be irritating to your skin, so it is best to thoroughly clean and let your skin breathe at night.) That's it! Wasn't so bad, right? Sleep tight.

## SUNDAY

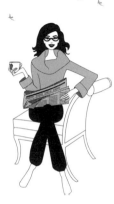

Good morning! Relax and enjoy your Sunday-morning ritual. Make a plan to go somewhere today. Make a date with the girls for brunch and shopping, or go for lunch and a stroll with your man. Just have an excuse to get out of the house so you can try out a daytime makeup look!

You're already an old pro. Last night you got comfortable

## DIY FACE MASKS FOR ALL SKIN TYPES

Egg white and yogurt mask: **2 egg whites and 2 tablespoons plain yogurt**

Banana mask: **½ banana, 1 tablespoon orange juice, and 1 tablespoon honey**

Coffee and cocoa mask: **4 tablespoons finely ground espresso or coffee beans; 4 tablespoons unsweetened cocoa powder; 8 tablespoons either whole milk, plain yogurt, almond milk, or coconut milk; 2 tablespoons honey**

Pumpkin mask: **½ cup fresh pumpkin pulp, 2 eggs, 2 teaspoons almond milk, 1 teaspoon honey**

with your new makeup tools and makeup supplies, so finding a daytime look or two will be a piece of cake. Your daytime look can simply be a lighter version of your nighttime one. Once you know how to apply your makeup, you can easily tone it down for day or spruce it up for a night out. There is nothing wrong with playing around and having fun. Maybe during the day you want nothing but a little mascara, blush, and lip gloss: whatever it is that gives you that little kick of feeling pretty.

**Remember, less is more.** You don't want to walk outside on Sunday morning and look like you just got home from a nightclub. Spend some time and figure out your best daytime look. Start with less makeup than you usually wear and only add if you feel you really need it. If mascara, blush, and lip gloss aren't enough, add a little eyeliner to the mix, or maybe go for a stronger lip. You'll know what feels right and looks good. There's no need to overdo it. Especially now that you have started your skin care regimen, your skin will be glowing all on its own.

**It's time for a last lesson in skin care.** Ready? The final step is to exfoliate and use a mask to remove impurities and cleanse your skin thoroughly. We recommend this routine once per week (a good time is Sunday evening) to keep your skin fresh and glowing.

Wash your face and neck with cleanser, then use an exfoliating scrub on your face and neck. (If you have sensitive skin, you should have a gentle scrub—nothing harsh.) Finally, apply a face mask. There are plenty of great options for masks out there, but we also like to make our own.

Depending on the package directions for your mask, you'll probably wear it for 10 to 20 minutes. Use this time to relax! Find something to watch or read. Or take a bath and let the mask do its work. If you are already in the bath, you might want to wash off the mask in the shower. Even if you aren't bathing, you might enjoy washing off the mask in the shower. Otherwise, remove it with a warm washcloth. The next step is to apply toner, if that's on your list, and then moisturizer. That wasn't so bad, was it? Your skin should feel and look great!

**Maintain your new beauty routine.** We're sure you want to keep up feeling and looking fabulous, so here's a quick rundown of what you need to do. Today, commit to your beauty routine. In 21 short days, you will have a new habit!

## BEAUTY CHECKLIST

**Morning:** Wash, tone, and moisturize your face and apply a daytime makeup look.

**Evening:** If going out, spruce up makeup with an evening look.

**Night:** Remove eye makeup, then wash, tone, and moisturize your face.

Two or three times per week (or as needed), exfoliate your face. (The easiest thing to do is to keep your exfoliator in the shower, so it is available and easy.)

Once a week, use a face mask. Make this a ritual. Sunday is the perfect day for this habit, but if you know you are always home on Wednesdays, that's fine, too.

Just give yourself 5 to 10 extra minutes in the morning and the same at night. Once a week, give yourself that extra half hour to exfoliate and apply the mask. You know you deserve it—and your skin will thank you!

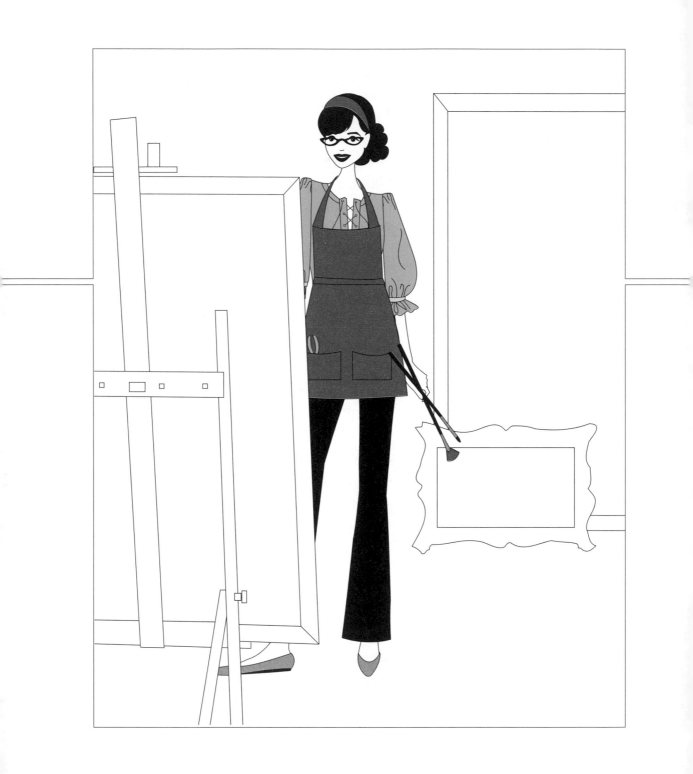

# Chapter Four
## Activity Makeover

Do you find that during your snippets of free time, for lack of anything better to do, you end up watching TV or reading a celebrity gossip magazine? Are there so many things you wish you were doing instead, but you haven't had the time or (in truth) energy to devote to learning something new? Are there things you would like to try but have put them out of your mind as activities you will get to when the kids grow up or when you retire?

Well, there is no time like the present! In fact, this very weekend. Don't waste another minute feeling unfulfilled or bored. Give yourself this weekend to learn a new hobby or get reacquainted with an old one. Maybe there is a skill you have always dreamed of achieving yet never learned how. Or maybe there is a hobby you had when you were younger, but you have gotten so out of the habit that you're not sure you remember how to do it.

This is your life. We want you to live it to the fullest. You deserve it. You are so busy giving to your family, your boss, your clients, whoever you deal with on a daily basis. Now take this weekend and give a little something back to yourself!

# ☾ FRIDAY NIGHT

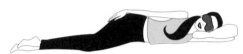

As you ease into your weekend, take time tonight to relax and push pause on your life. Make yourself a healthy, yummy dinner. Then compile a list of all the things you have always wanted to learn.

**What's on your wish list?** There are so many things to choose from! Have you always wanted to draw or paint? Maybe pottery intrigues you. Or knitting, sewing, jewelry making, gardening, photography, playing the piano (or any other instrument), writing, or cooking. Anything that gives you a creative outlet will be stimulating and rewarding.

Perhaps you have friends who would love to join you in a quest for a new and fun hobby. There are things you can do as pairs or groups—playing chess or card games. Even mahjong is no longer just for the elderly retired set anymore. It seems to be all the rage among young suburban moms!

Not to get too far ahead of ourselves, but you would be amazed at how many businesses developed from hobbies. There are countless stories about women (and men!) who initially made things for themselves (jewelry, clothing, cupcakes). Then word got out and people started asking to buy their goods, and, sure enough, a business was born. (We are not implying that you give up your day job yet! Rather, we just want you to know the endless possibilities of doing something you enjoy.)

There may be several activities you've always wanted to try. That's fantastic. Once you start the first hobby, you may be motivated to keep learning and incorporating more fun hobbies into your repertoire. This weekend, though, we would love for you to pick your number-one activity goal and focus on that. You want to be able to devote time, especially in the beginning and particularly this weekend, to developing the skills and getting the supplies you need to make this hobby part of every day or at least every week!

Some things to consider when picking your hobby:

*Lifestyle.* Think about your choices and your lifestyle. If you are at home a lot, maybe painting or practicing an instrument is realistic for you. If you are constantly on the go, find a hobby with easily totable supplies, like knitting, sketching, or photography.

*Budget.* Some hobbies require expensive supplies (a piano or another musical instrument, for example), while others are practically free (some drawing pencils and a sketch pad). The other part of the equation is how you will learn. Private lessons are pricier than learning from a book or an online video. Taking a single class falls somewhere in the middle.

> ## TOP 10 HOBBIES THAT WON'T BREAK THE BANK
>
> 1. Cooking/baking
> 2. Creating music playlists
> 3. Drawing
> 4. Flower arranging
> 5. Jewelry making
> 6. Knitting
> 7. Playing cards/games/chess
> 8. Sewing
> 9. Singing
> 10. Writing/journaling/blogging

If you truly want to learn something, and the supplies and lessons cost more than you had hoped to spend, don't be discouraged. These days, you can learn almost anything on the computer or your smartphone! There is an app (or online video tutorial) for pretty much everything. Along with the apps, there are even corresponding gadgets that you can connect to your iPhone or iPad that will have you playing the piano or guitar without actually touching a piano or guitar. Your options are limitless. It's about being a little creative in finding a way to learn that fits into your budget comfortably. Once you see that you are really learning and loving it, maybe saving up for an actual instrument and lessons will become a priority for you.

*Space.* This weekend is all about you, but you might share your home with others. If you live with a partner and/or kids, find a space at home that you can set up as your "hobby station." Even if you live alone, giving yourself a separate, dedicated space is ideal. You may not need a lot of room if you are writing, sketching, or knitting, but if you are painting, practicing a musical instrument, making clothes on a sewing machine, or baking or cooking up a storm, make sure you have the space to work and that it's a space that you can keep clean and available. You always want your home to look tidy and uncluttered and pretty, but you also want your hobby supplies to be easily accessible. If you have to pack up and put away equipment and supplies after every use, you'll be less tempted to sit down for 10 minutes and play. The goal is for you to participate as much as you can and would like, so convenience is key.

*Time.* You'll need an hour, or an hour and a half, a week for some sort of lesson, whether it is a private tutorial, a class, or self-instruction from a guidebook. You'll also need practice time throughout the week. Be realistic about how much time you can devote. Most hobbies, once you get the hang of them, can easily be picked up and put down throughout the day or the week and don't require long stretches of time to participate. You can knit for 10 minutes and see results, but you might want to give yourself an hour or two to play cards with your friends. Practicing a musical instrument can be accomplished in 30-minute slots. When you get into the groove of painting or sketching, you may decide to extend your sessions. Available free time should not be the biggest factor in your decision, however, as whatever time you can provide will keep you learning, growing, and enjoying. The more you relish your hobby, the more hours you will want to spend on it. Don't let a fear of lack of time steer you away from an activity you are passionate about.

Sleep on your ideas, and we'll start the next step in the morning.

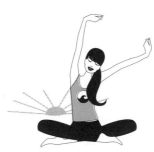

## SATURDAY MORNING

Have you selected your hobby? Great! Let's get started. Your hobby will fall into one of three categories: something you already know how to do, something you have no idea how to do and that requires private lessons or a class, or something that can be self-taught.

*Jill*      I recently took up a new hobby, and it has changed my life. Two years ago, my friend Shawn took me on a surfing lesson with a guy we call "Mr. Adventure"! I mean, how can you go wrong with a name like that? His real name is Orion, and he introduced me to surfing and paddleboarding. I work 6 days a week (sometimes 7), and until recently, I never had an adult hobby. I am so grateful for my new interest. It is the only time I am without my BlackBerry and able to relax. I've realized two things as I've gotten older: It is harder to make new friends, and it is harder to find something you are truly passionate about. I have been fortunate to find both. (I met my co-author 6 years ago, and she is like a sister to me.)

*Dana*      It's funny, I consider myself a creative person, but for whatever reason, I do not enjoy knitting, sewing, cooking, or playing the piano. And believe me, I have tried them all! (Luckily for me, my mom and sister are knitters, sewers, and awesome cooks, so you know where I go when I need something in those departments!) However, I do enjoy fashion, music, and eating. So instead of actually making clothing or playing a musical instrument, my hobbies are putting fun outfits together for myself and friends and making music playlists and CDs for my friends and especially my niece. I also love to decorate, so I consider interior design a hobby, too. Every time I move, or every few years or so, I love to transform my home. Writing and photography are my other favorite pastimes. I am a new and huge fan of sharing my favorite shots on Instagram!

If you already know how to do your hobby, you are ahead of the game. Sit tight; we will get to your next step shortly. On the other hand, if you have some familiarity with your hobby but are not proficient, or you have not reached the level of skill you like, or you just need a little brushup because it's been a long while, read on.

If your hobby is something you have no idea how to do or have never done before, let's get you into lessons or a class. Take this morning for online research or to talk with friends currently learning the subject. The goal is to find a great private teacher or a class that you can register for to begin instruction.

Something like playing an instrument may be better learned with one-on-one instruction (although private sessions are not necessary), whereas knitting, sewing, pottery, drawing, painting, cooking, photography, and even writing can be done (and will probably be a lot more fun) in a classroom setting. A class will be easier on your budget than private lessons, but personal instruction can definitely be worth the investment. Learning a new skill or hobby is something of great value, and if you can afford lessons, go for it.

Incredibly, some people have a knack for teaching themselves new skills, and others were born with certain abilities and talents. Get them in the kitchen and they can improvise and make a delicious meal; hand someone a guitar and she is naturally able to play a tune; or give someone else a sketchbook and he is able to draw the most beautiful picture. These are exceptions, for sure, but it can happen. If you fall into that category, lucky you! If not, some people—and you may be one—can still be self-taught. Tons of books, articles, and apps on the market can teach you how to teach yourself almost anything if you prefer self-instruction to attending a class. This option is also perfect for those with time or budget con-straints. You can carve out time when it fits your schedule rather than have to plan around a class offering, and the price for self-instruction is definitely right.

With all your options before you, now it's time to pick your method of learning. You might want to attend a class just for the fun of it. You might make new friends while developing a new skill. And it helps to have the aid, feedback, and motiva-tion of a teacher or fellow students.

The class you want to take may not be held today, or even this weekend, but regardless, this is your activity weekend and you are starting your hobby *today*. If you are going to take a class or work with a teacher, register or make your first appointment now so that you have a solid plan for the first lesson this coming week.

If you are going to learn from a book or an app or online instruction, download it now. If you prefer to peruse the bookstore and leaf through instruction manuals and guides to find one that resonates with you, that will be your first stop this afternoon.

And if you are all set with the know-how and you just need to get back in the game, please rejoin us here.

The type of hobby you choose will determine what kind of space you need. Identify that space in your home before you shop for supplies. If you plan to draw or paint, you will need at least an empty corner with some nice light to dedicate to this craft. If you intend to play an instrument, you will also need some space (preferably your own room, if you have it, but that's not necessary). If you wish to cook, make sure your kitchen is tidy and can accommodate any new gadgets or utensils you will need. If you desire to knit, or write, or anything else that doesn't require much space, you are probably all set.

Relax, have a little lunch, and get excited to go shopping for supplies!

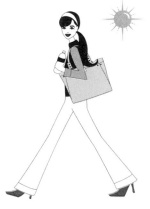 ## SATURDAY AFTERNOON

If you need to hit the bookstore, head there first. Pick up a how-to guide or two (or a few recipe books) and maybe a magazine or two about your new hobby. These references are always handy and definitely interesting, even if you are taking a class or getting private instruction. It never hurts to read up and get more information when you are learning something new. You might find someone researching the same topic who has words of wisdom.

Your next stop will be to gather the supplies you need to get started. This may mean a visit to a specialty store, an art supply store, or an all-purpose store like Target.

A musical hobby can be a big financial investment on every level, including lessons and the instrument itself. We are all for this, but you need to seriously commit to learning before you expend the cash. Perhaps you already have a piano in your living room or you've had a guitar since you were young. If so, fantastic! Your next steps will be to get it tuned up and buy some sheet music. If you don't want to follow the traditional lessons route and instead want to learn on your iPad or other device, get whatever electronic gadget you need to practice on, and research the apps to find the best instructional series.

The art supply store will have everything you need to start painting or drawing: paints, brushes, pencils, sketch pads, canvases, and an easel to set up at home. An arts and crafts store offers supplies to start playing around with jewelry design or any other crafts you would like to create. Or find a dedicated jewelry crafting store stocked with beads, strings, and clasps, or a specialty store for whatever supplies your hobby requires.

The grocery store and home stores like Bed Bath & Beyond, Williams-Sonoma, and Target carry any needed cooking and baking supplies, utensils, and kitchenware. Stock up on ingredients for some of the recipes you will want to learn, and maybe invest in an apron!

Hit the yarn or fabric store, or both, to purchase what you need to knit or sew. For knitting, get yourself needles in a variety of sizes and a few skeins of yarn. For sewing, invest in fabric and thread and, if you don't have one already, a sewing machine. This machine is a big expense, so know that you are committing to your new hobby when you make this purchase.

If you want to write, pick out some special supplies to make the words flow and sing. Perhaps you want to try writing with a new fountain pen in a bound journal with beautiful paper. If you prefer to type on the computer, that's fine, too. You don't need a brand-new laptop unless you really want to treat yourself!

You may already have all the supplies you need if snapping photos is your new hobby. You can do this with just your smartphone! If you want to get a little fancy and have a separate camera to make it official, you can find this at any camera or electronics shop.

You'll find all the supplies you need for some hobbies, like pottery, in the

*Jill* *Paddleboarding is obviously not a hobby I can do in my living room, so I have to find time in my schedule and make this activity part of my routine to ensure I keep up with it. I started doing these creative excursions with my trainer, Orion, three times a week. (Picture me on the beach running with a parachute strapped to my back. And, yes, Orion provides all of these supplies. I do not store a paddleboard and parachute in my hall closet!) We do beach workouts that involve everything from digging in the sand to passing a water bottle to a friend while doing situps. Only after that warmup is finished do we paddleboard back to our starting point. I love my new hobby. I actually plan vacations around paddleboarding. It is nice to be passionate about something that is just plain fun. I'm lucky I found something I love to do (other than work)!*

*Dana* *My dad taught himself to play the guitar and the drums. Mind you, the drums take up a bit of room, but, nevertheless, he found the space and set them up in his home office. He also found the time. Growing up, my sister and I would always hear him practicing. I think this was a major escape and stress relief for him. My friend Lance's hobby is painting. He has his easel set up in his dining area. Even with all the canvases, it still looks organized and beautiful in his apartment. It is art, after all! No matter how busy you are or how little space you have, you can always make a hobby work.*

classroom or studio. We don't expect you to install a kiln at your house (but you can rent the movie *Ghost* to watch tonight and get inspired!).

**Set up your dedicated space.** Once you have your supplies, go home and set up the area or room you have designated as your hobby station. You'll be devoting time and attention to your new hobby, so make it feel important and a priority. Once the station is set up, and once you get the hang of your new hobby, you will be amazed at how easy it is to sneak in 10 minutes here or 30 minutes there on your new activity. That's why it's so crucial that you get yourself sorted this weekend. Once you are in motion, you will find that practicing your new skill becomes addictive and a welcome escape from your everyday stresses.

**Get creative and play!** Now that you have set up your easel, your kitchen, your sewing machine, your musical instrument, your desk, or any other area you have designated as your hobby station, dive in! You may feel a bit overwhelmed, and your lessons may not start until the coming week, but regardless, you can still have a little fun and begin the habit of practicing your hobby rather than turning on the TV.

If you have chosen something that requires a classroom setting, because it is not feasible to do at home, such as pottery, you can still participate today. Do a little research online to find a nearby shop or studio that will let you get started today. A popular chain of pottery studios is Color Me Mine. You make whatever you like in its workroom and leave the mess behind. Even if you are crafting in an outside facility, however, make sure you have space in your home to proudly display everything you've made.

If you are set up at home, familiarize yourself with your new station and supplies. Go ahead, paint something—anything! It doesn't have to be perfect, and it doesn't even need to look like something. The point is to make the experience fun and creative for you. Or go ahead, cook or bake something. Prepare a meal for yourself, for you and your partner, or for friends. Bake a cake for someone's birthday or cookies to take into the office next week. Just play. Nothing bad will happen if your concoction doesn't look like something out of *Martha Stewart Living* magazine. Sewing? Try something simple, like a pillow. Knitting? Start a

*Jill* *As a reporter for the Knicks, I work on a lot of Sundays. The way I look at it, sometimes Sundays are my Mondays. I bet many of you feel the same way if your job is not conventional or you have kids whose activities take up your weekends. So I make sure that I find other times to play at my hobbies—times where I can put down my iPad, BlackBerry, or whatever and just relax and let loose.*

*Dana* *I do my best writing in the morning. In the middle of the night, when the rest of the world is quiet, my mind whirls with things I want to say. Even while I'm sleeping, I will construct whole paragraphs in my head. Writing these down when I first get up is almost a necessity. It is a huge relief to be able to journal or write a letter and get my ideas down on paper. The minute I am able to express myself in this way, my mind stops racing, and I feel lighter, accomplished, productive, creative, and stress free.*

scarf. It doesn't matter what it is. Go for it! Sit at the piano and play some scales or let your fingers get familiar with the keys. Simply immerse yourself in your new hobby and savor the excitement to learn. Sit at your desk or curl up in a chair and journal about your day or write a long letter to an old friend. Call some friends and organize a card game or mahjong for tomorrow. Yes, you will be practicing your new hobby tomorrow, too!

This is your time, your weekend. We know you probably never get this kind of free time to devote to anything that is purely fun and self-enriching, so take advantage. No guilt here. It is your chance to feel like a kid again. If you have children, you watch them learning and growing and experimenting all the time. Now it's your turn! So take this afternoon to play. Take as long as you like. You may get so caught up that you forget where you are and what time it is. Enjoy it! You deserve it.

When you are done for the day, clean up. Keep your new hobby station in order. Especially if you live with a partner and kids, you want them to respect your new space as much as you respect theirs. Have a relaxing night. We hope you are looking forward to a little more playtime tomorrow.

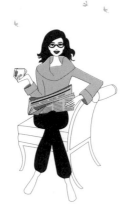

# SUNDAY

To develop the habit of keeping up with your new hobby, find time to practice and play today, too. Maybe you are in the middle of a project from yesterday, maybe you want to start from scratch this morning, or maybe before you play this afternoon, you want to read about your hobby to learn or get tips before you start formal instruction.

If your instruction is going to be solely from books or articles or from an app, definitely take the time today to read and teach yourself the first lesson. The goal is to get you truly invested this weekend so that you have a strong commitment to learning and practicing your new hobby.

If you are not able to take your first lesson because you are waiting for class or an appointment with your teacher, just continue to mess around a bit until you start your formal training this week. You'll be amazed what you can create without even being in a class.

Here's the other thing you need to sort out today: setting aside time in your busy week to play and practice at your hobby. Especially if you are learning something new, like how to play a musical instrument, you will need practice time besides your lessons to stay on track and see results.

If you have signed up for a class or private lessons, obviously, that time is already allotted for your hobby. Likely this instruction will be once a week. If you haven't signed up for a class, pick a workable time slot for you to give yourself a weekly lesson. Find an hour or an hour and a half that you can consider yourself to be "in class."

Class, course, private instruction, or self-instruction—regardless of your approach, you need to find some time to practice on your own in the coming days. Hopefully, you truly love this new hobby and are excited to learn and practice. If you can devote a half hour just two or even three times per week, that would be ideal. Even if you sneak in 15 minutes here and there, you're in good shape. You can pick up your knitting needles for 5 minutes in the car while you are waiting to collect your kids from school and still be working toward your goal of making your first scarf or whatever you choose. The trick is to keep up with your hobby. Remember, it takes just 21 days to form a habit. In the next 3 crucial weeks, if you practice a little bit every day, or a little more every other day, fantastic. Truly, this makeover is for you—for your stress relief, your enrichment, and your enjoyment. Good luck and have fun!

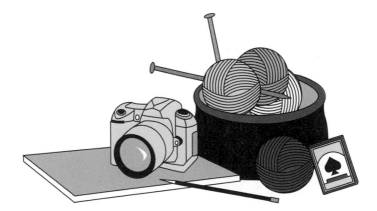

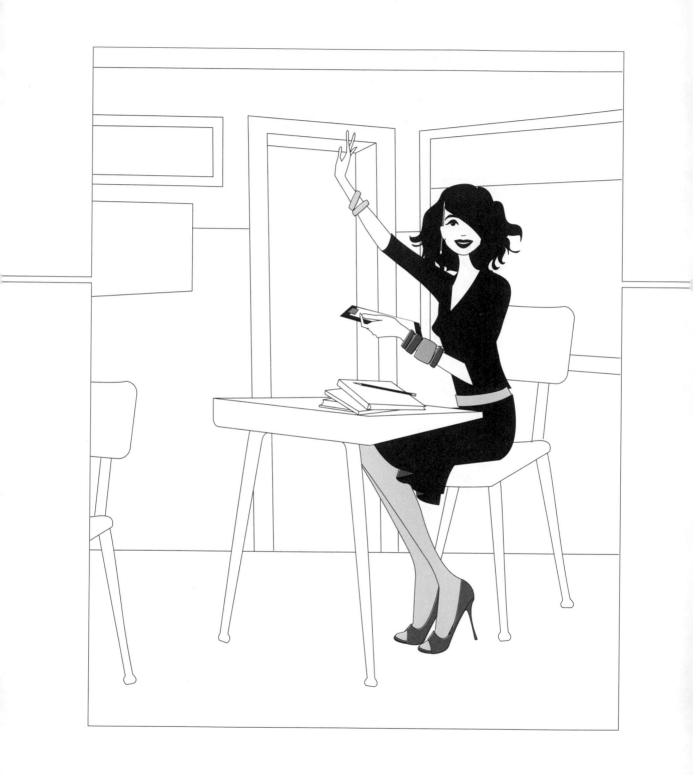

# Chapter Five

# Brain Makeover

Has it been a while, a long while maybe, since you've done anything to stimulate your brain? Have you given up not only reading challenging books but reading—period? Are you amazed at what your kids are learning in school and at how little recollection you have of what you learned at the same age?

Our brains need constant nourishment to stay sharp. According to a study by the Franklin Institute, most age-related losses in memory or motor skills are a result of physical inactivity and lack of mental exercise and stimulation. Once we finish school, get jobs, and start our adult lives, we think we're home free, but the reality is that learning is something we can—and should—do our entire lives. The same study found that our brains are able to rewire and adapt, even in old age. So use it—don't lose it!—because the feeling of pride and accomplishment is something you can attain at any age.

We know you're very busy with work, with family, with running a household and just getting through the day. But wouldn't it be great to *celebrate* the day and not just get through it? It's so easy to zone out in front of the TV or flip through a gossip magazine at the nail salon. Well, guess what? It's just as easy to pick up a classic novel that you've never read or work on a crossword puzzle!

You may or may not have enjoyed school, but it's your chance as an adult to make learning fun. You are free to learn whatever you like, with no pressure about grades or college acceptances. Taking a class to learn a new subject or to brush up on a topic you have nearly forgotten is a challenge you can give yourself purely for the joy of learning, acquiring a skill, and expanding your knowledge. If you hated math, no one will ever force you to take a math class again! But if you used to be pretty good at Spanish and are now totally out of practice, well . . .

This weekend is all about *you*—finding something to challenge your mind, starting to work toward your goal, and learning how to prioritize your brain makeover in your busy schedule.

## ( FRIDAY NIGHT

Everyone (we hope!) has a list of things, either written down or in their mind's eye, that they hope to accomplish at some point. When is "some point"? Truthfully, our lives get so busy that we have to make a point of making some point, *now*. This is why you are taking this weekend: to make your priorities come to fruition.

**It's not too late to learn something new.** This evening, as you ease into the weekend, reflect on all the things you wish you had learned or accomplished, whether in school or elsewhere. UCLA brain researcher Gary Small says our complex reasoning skills improve as we reach middle age, thanks to a process called "myelination." (Myelin is the insulation wrapped around nerve cells that speeds up the travel time of information from brain cell to brain cell.) Myelination doesn't reach its peak until middle age—which means most of us can look forward to reasoning and anticipating problems even better than we do now. You are capable and smart, and now you are giving yourself the opportunity to take advantage of the brain's ability to improve. What an incredible gift to give yourself—and one you deserve.

As we've said before, when you feel satisfied, challenged, accomplished, and refreshed, everyone around you appreciates the new you, too. These positive feelings not only affect how you operate in the world, but they also energize everyone you come in contact with. This is why we're sure that whoever helps you to take care of your usual duties—kids, house, husband, etc.—while you pursue your brain-building interests will be more than happy to continue the support, so that you can relax and enjoy this weekend makeover guilt free.

**Get excited to go back to school.** If you haven't thought about your to-learn list, take the time now. You have all evening. Perhaps learning a language is intriguing. This could mean brushing up and expanding on the Spanish or French you took in high school or, if you are proficient in a second language, adding a third one to your repertoire, such as Italian or Chinese or Japanese. Go for it!

Perhaps you have always wanted to take a business, real estate, or law course. You don't have to go for a degree to satisfy your curiosity and gather information that might be useful in your life or your work. It's amazing how empowering it feels to learn simply because you have the desire and the interest, not because you have to. If you end up wanting to complete a college degree or go for a postgraduate diploma, even better! What an accomplishment that will be!

Or your mind challenge could be something like reading (or rereading) the classics. There's a reason certain books are considered classics—because they are, well, classic. But you don't have to read *War and Peace*. Simply starting to read again is great brain stimulation. We are on technology sensory overload: With so many TV shows, DVR programs, and Web sites, who makes time to read anymore? We spend almost 3 hours a day watching TV, according to the Bureau of Labor Statistic's American Time Use Survey—3½ hours if you don't have kids.

Reading is a challenge you can do on your own, but if you need companions to keep you on track, taking a literature course is a great treat. Another fun, social way to stay on top of your reading is to start a book club with friends. This way you will have deadlines, discussions, and friends to help out with your reading list.

**Play games!** Crossword puzzles and other challenges like word scrambles and

*Jill* I went to the University of Michigan and majored in communications. I always knew I wanted to go into television, so I took film and video courses and then a variety of other classes. The one thing I regret not doing is taking as many languages as possible. My mother is a Spanish and French teacher, and the fact that I can't speak either language fluently is awful. I speak enough to get around when I travel, but if I had to do my schooling over again, I would master as many languages as possible. I have recently decided to take up French. My mom and I meet once a week for lunch, and I take an hour lesson with her. It feels great to be a student again.

*Dana* I always wanted to speak another language. Originally, I planned to take French in school, but I ended up taking Spanish through college. (Thanks, Mom.) After I graduated, I signed up for two consecutive classes in French at the Alliance Française. Postcollege, I have also taken Spanish classes. I can get by in Spanish but not at all in French. Several friends speak Spanish fluently, and I am soooooo jealous. I took literature classes in school, too, but of course there were classic books and authors I never read. So I make a point to read those that I missed, and I continue to be a voracious reader. When I lived in LA, I started a book club with several girlfriends. It definitely kept me on top of my game and on deadline, and it was a blast. We each hosted dinners in the theme of whatever the book was for that month, and we switched up the genre every time. I still consult my book club friends for reading suggestions. And actually, I think it's time to look into another language class!

Sudoku will keep your intellect sharp, and these are games you can pick up and put down whenever you have a spare couple of minutes. One study at Rush University Medical Center in Chicago tracked the mental activity of elderly participants. The study found that keeping mentally fit through activities like reading and doing puzzles was a good way to preserve memory as we age. The more puzzles you do, the better you will get. Keep challenging yourself with more difficult crossword puzzles as you continue improving until you can do the crossword in the Sunday *New York Times* in pen!

Overall, the more you read, the more languages you know, and the more knowledge you have on a variety of subjects, the more you'll improve conversationally, socially, and culturally—not to mention the improved brain function. Challenging yourself intellectually will have a payoff in more than one department!

Remember, this makeover challenge is for you to enjoy. It shouldn't be overwhelming or dreadful. No one is forcing you to go back to school, but tapping a natural desire to learn and expand your mind is healthy. Patricia McKinley of McGill University found that older adults who learned the Argentine tango, which combines social interaction with physical exercise and mental challenge (hey, you try remembering all of those steps!), had better cognition and were better able to perform day-to-day tasks.

Pick something that intrigues, stimulates, or inspires you. Write down your goal if that will help you feel confident that you'll achieve it. Now, get a good night's sleep so you're well rested and ready to go in the morning.

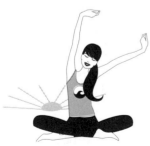

## SATURDAY MORNING

This morning, we work toward your goal. No rush; this is your weekend to make over your mind. Your only agenda is to put your challenge into action.

The following factors should not make or break your decision regarding your challenge choice or how you will go about achieving your goal, but they can help you refine your goal:

## Purpose

Are you pursuing this goal as a means to further your business or to foster your personal growth and knowledge? Either purpose, or both, is correct and amazing. Knowing the underlying reason might help you allocate your budget and time. If you are taking a course to bolster your business skills, the cost of the class may be tax deductible, and you might thus be able to justify investing more time.

## Personality

You know yourself well enough to recognize that you either have the discipline to teach or push yourself or that you do better when you have a teacher or a group motivating you and keeping you on track toward your goal. If you can teach yourself, fantastic. If you know that will never happen, prepare to sign up for a formal class, get tutoring, or work with a group.

## Budget

Figure out what is financially viable for you. There are several ways to reach your goal: registering for an official class, teaching or motivating yourself with guide-books or by listening to CDs, or learning with friends. With all the online courses available these days, you will probably be able to find a class you can afford, even if it is not in a traditional classroom setting. So don't be immediately dissuaded by cost. Finding a budget-friendly course simply entails a bit of research.

## Time

Learning a new language or taking a business class will require a larger time investment than, say, reading a novel or working on a crossword puzzle. So time is certainly a factor to consider. But if you really want to learn something that requires classroom hours and probably homework, you'll have to find the time. If the subject interests and challenges you, it is worth the time investment.

Now that you've decided on your goal, let's take action. Whether or not you can start your class or lessons today is not as important as signing up for it and

*Jill*    I believe in doing anything that will keep me off my Blackberry, iPhone, or any of my other devices. I think it is important to leave your electronics alone and go back to the basics. I still read the newspapers that arrive at my door (not on the computer) and always have a book at my bedside. I try to read at least a chapter before I go to bed at night of everything from Emily Giffin to Deepak Chopra to the latest biography on bookstands. Reading keeps your mind active no matter what the subject.

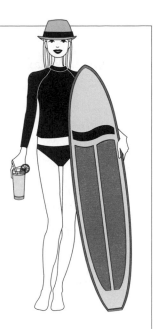

*Dana*    I still read books—yes, "real" books. Someone saw me in my elevator recently with a package from Amazon, and he asked, "People still read actual books?" I said, "Yes!" (I know I'm a little behind the times, but I didn't realize it was that uncommon.) I spend a lot of time on the computer, so when I am on a plane or at the beach, and when I crawl into bed at night, I prefer to be as far away from anything electronic as I can get. Funnily enough, I do have an unopened Kindle sitting in my closet. Truth be told, I am a little intimidated, but I should try it—at least when I think of all the trees that go into making printed books!

## 10 CLASSIC NOVELS NOT TO BE MISSED

1. *Gone with the Wind,* by Margaret Mitchell

2. *The Great Gatsby,* by F. Scott Fitzgerald

3. *Little Women,* by Louisa May Alcott

4. *The Odyssey,* by Homer

5. *On the Road,* by Jack Kerouac

6. *Pride and Prejudice,* by Jane Austen

7. *The Sun Also Rises,* by Ernest Hemingway

8. *Tess of the D'urbervilles,* by Thomas Hardy

9. *To Kill a Mockingbird,* by Harper Lee

10. *Tom Jones,* by Henry Fielding

getting whatever supplies you need to get psyched and ready to learn. Today, we want you immersed in your challenge.

**Prepare for your new education.** If you are going to take a class, either at a school facility or online, register now. If you are taking a language, being in a classroom setting to practice speaking with other students and a teacher is key. If you are taking business, real estate, law, or any subject of that nature, an online class will probably suffice. However, some people like the feeling of sitting in a classroom. Especially if your job has you isolated in front of the computer all day, it might be a nice change of pace to get into a new setting and meet new people.

If you plan to teach yourself either by reading books or listening to CDs, browse around online to see what materials are available. If you use a Kindle, an iPad, or a laptop, download your learning tools now. If not, make a list of what you are going to buy at the bookstore today.

If you are going to learn with friends (which can not only be motivating but also provides quality time with your pals), set a plan. A great idea if friends also want to brush up on their Spanish, for example, is to hire a private tutor and split the fee. This way, the learning will cost less, you will have people to practice with, and you can create your own classroom environment—maybe you even meet at a tapas bar for lessons or practice sessions without the teacher.

If your challenge is to start reading again, or to read all those classic novels you never finished, decide if you will meet this goal on your own or if you want to recruit friends for a book club. Make a list of must-reads and buy at least three books to get you started today. You can download the books onto your electronic device or order bound copies online if you love the feel of a physical book. Better yet, pay a visit to your local library and borrow books for free! Just to make sure you get started today. If you don't download your first book, you should get it at your local bookstore or from the library this afternoon. Having those must-reads at the ready will help you commit to your goal. Depending on the books' lengths and your available time, if you average one book per week, you will make it to the 21-day habit-forming finish line when you complete those first three. (Tip: Before you start the last book, order another three!)

If you are going to start or join a book club, reach out to friends who love to read or who currently belong to a book club. (If you are new in town or don't know other avid readers, check out your local library for book club suggestions. Or research online at sites such as www.goodreads.com or www.shelfari.com to connect with other readers.) Set your first meeting date and pick your first book, or get on board with the book the club has already picked.

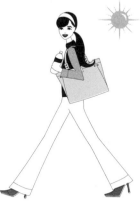

## SATURDAY AFTERNOON

There's no time like the present to get in the mood to learn. If you haven't downloaded everything you need, let's get to the store to browse around. Buy a novel to start today. Purchase (or download) music CDs or audio learning CDs in the language you will be studying. Get a workbook that will aid you in your classroom study or that you will use to teach yourself. Buy a bunch of crossword puzzle workbooks (or your choice of word-challenging games) or pick up today's newspaper to see how far you get with its puzzle. Pick up new school supplies, too. Treat yourself to a new notebook and a new pen. Remember how much fun shopping for school supplies was when you were a kid?

**Class is in session.** Once you are stocked with supplies, registered for class, or scheduled for your first book club meeting, it's time to introduce yourself to your

*Jill* *I read the papers every morning. Five papers, cover to cover. They arrive at my doorstep—no iPad version for me. The one thing I never miss? The word jumble! I come from a long line of "jumblers," and every morning I take the mixed-up letters and put them in the proper sequence. If I can't solve one? I call my father. He always gets 'em. The jumble revs up my mind. What's your game?*

*Dana* *My mother and grandmother are always reading. My mom is a crossword fanatic, and my grandmother (at 93 years old) does not feel her day is complete if she hasn't solved the word scramble in the paper. Their constant reading and having books around were huge influences on me.*

subject. This afternoon is like the first day back at school. You don't have to devote the whole day to your study, by any means, but take advantage of this weekend's goal to get on track.

If you are starting a book, whether you have joined a book club or not, set aside time this afternoon to curl up in your favorite spot and just read. Get absorbed enough in your book that you are vested in the story line and the characters to ensure that you will continue to make time to keep reading.

If crosswords or other mind-challenging games and puzzles are your choice, find some time and a cozy corner to exercise your brain.

If learning or refreshing a language is your goal, start to incorporate basic words and phrases like *hello, goodbye, how are you,* and *thank you* into your daily routine. Speak them to your partner, your kids, or just to yourself! Using the language, even at a basic level, will start you thinking in that language and motivate you to learn more.

Another fun tool is to listen to music in the language you'd like to learn. Instead of listening to the same old playlist on your iPod or the radio, put on foreign language CDs or downloads and get immersed in the culture. Keep some in your car, too. You may learn a language more like a native speaker by getting out of the classroom and immersing yourself in the culture, according to brain studies by researchers at Georgetown University Medical Center. "Only the immersion training led to full native-like brain processing of grammar," says Michael Ullman, a professor of neuroscience and the studies' senior investigator.

You may get so inspired by your language learning that you'll want to eat at an Italian, Spanish, Mexican, Chinese, Japanese, or [*fill in the cuisine here*] restaurant for dinner tonight. Before you go out, look up a couple of phrases and teach yourself how to order your favorite dish in that language.

If your plan is to go back to school for professional classes (business, real estate, law, etc.), you can get in the game today, too. Leaf through any reading materials you purchased today and put your mind in that mode. If you are going to teach yourself a subject, give yourself lesson one. Break open your new textbook and start at the beginning. You will need self-discipline if you are not attending a scheduled class, so it is important that you get your feet wet today while you have the weekend dedicated to this goal.

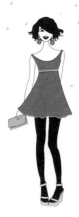

## SATURDAY NIGHT

Tonight, reward your hard work with a nice, relaxing dinner. Tell your companions about your goal. When you tell people what you hope to accomplish, they will get right on board to support you. Talk about the book you started today, practice ordering dinner in the language you are starting to learn, or tell people why you are choosing to go back to school (or take a class) on this particular subject.

It's finally time for bed. If you started a book earlier, you might enjoy reading another chapter before you drift off to sleep. The benefits of reading before sleep began when you were a child enjoying bedtime stories. One study from Stony Brook University School of Medicine shows that regular use of bedtime routines like reading may have a lasting, positive benefit for children's sleep duration and cognitive development.

Those of you whose chosen activities (language learning, professional development) require a bit more concentration, stimulation, and time allotment might want to leave reading those textbooks until tomorrow. Good job today. Sleep well.

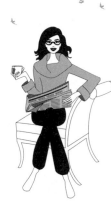

# SUNDAY

Today, we take another step toward a more active brain. Let's get further immersed in learning and make a plan to incorporate time in your busy week to work toward your goal.

**Read whenever you can.** If you started a new book yesterday and it is on your nightstand, read another chapter or two this morning before you get out of bed. This is a most luxurious activity—one that we don't all get to do very often. Enjoy!

Make use of other free time during the day to continue reading. Hopefully, you are so engrossed in the story by now that you won't want to put it down. Tonight before you go to sleep will be another opportunity to dip into your book.

As you can see, incorporating reading (if this is your challenge of choice) is definitely one of the easier goals to squeeze into your life. There is really no excuse, as these days you can even read a book on your phone! Whether you are riding public transportation, waiting for your kids at school, or standing on line at the post office, you can always sneak in 10 minutes or another chapter! Get in the habit of making wise use of time, and you'll find that even if you can't set aside hours in your week, all these stolen moments will ultimately help you meet your goal. When you read, you change your brain forever—both physiologically and intellectually, according to Maryanne Wolf, Tufts University cognitive neuroscientist and child development expert.

If you joined a book group, today you will also need to plan for the once-a-month meeting. Yesterday, you put the first meeting date in your calendar, and somehow we think you will have no problem finding the time for this activity. If you read at every opportunity (while waiting for someone or in line at the store, etc.), we're sure that you will have time not only for your book club book but also for whatever else is on your master list of unread tomes.

**Play games!** You can sneak in a crossword puzzle, word scramble, or Sudoku at random opportune moments as well. These games are portable (whether on your phone or in small, easy-to-carry pads or books) and can be picked up, put down, and worked on in spurts. To get in the habit, devote some time today to thoroughly challenge yourself. Set aside a time block—that is, more than just a few moments grabbed while in line at the supermarket. You want to establish this challenge for yourself so that puzzle solving becomes second nature and your go-to activity.

Once you find yourself competing with yourself (in a good way, of course), you will not be able to put these games down. Take your games with you every day so that when you take a break at the office, or are waiting for a friend for lunch, you can improve your skills and get closer to finishing that Sunday *Times* puzzle or whatever your personal goal. You'll be surprised at how many opportunities present themselves in a day.

**Prepare for class.** Of course, learning a new language or taking a professional class requires a larger time-block commitment than developing the reading habit or challenging yourself with puzzles. These are lofty and important goals, however, and you can reach them with a little dedication and smart time management. Which is why today, and this weekend, is so crucial to getting you on track.

You have selected your method of learning—whether you signed up for a formal class, hired a private or group tutor, or committed to teaching yourself through guidebooks, audio CDs, or downloads. Regardless of your choice, today you will dedicate some time on your subject.

Waiting to take your first class or to meet with your tutor? Spend maybe an hour or so today to thumb through the books that you bought—either handbooks or the class's actual texts or workbooks. Taking a business or real estate class? Read those sections of the newspaper (if you do this already, great!) and get acquainted with the market and the lingo. Taking a language class? Listen again to music and leaf through fashion magazines in that language. Edith Piaf and French *Vogue* perhaps?

Mark your date book or calendar with time slots for studying or homework. If you are taking a class or studying with a tutor, you will likely meet once or twice a week for about an hour and a half each session. You will need to set aside some real time to concentrate and complete your work for the next class. Once you start the course, you will figure out what kind of time you need. Likely, you will need a couple additional hours every week. Decide if you will break that study time into an hour a day two or three times per week, or if you are going to devote solid time over the weekend. We suggest keeping up with your work throughout the week, if possible, especially at first. This approach is more beneficial because it keeps the lessons fresh in your mind, and you won't feel weighed down all in one sitting.

Teaching yourself? We're impressed! Yesterday you started with lesson one. Today, finish and/or review lesson one and do any work or writing or practice so that you "own" that lesson and feel prepared to tackle lesson two. We don't want you to feel overwhelmed, so you don't have to start lesson two today (unless, of course, you want to!). We really just want you to get in the groove. Accomplishing lesson one is huge. Making sure you own what you learned before moving on is key to success.

To keep up with lessons (if you aren't taking a formal scheduled class), you must schedule time in your week for lessons and any relevant practice work/homework. Set the goal of one lesson per week. Mark your calendar with a time slot for the actual lesson (allow at least an hour and a half) and a couple of shorter slots (maybe an hour each) to do your practice work. This is going to take some real discipline on your part, but we have total faith in you. As you start to see results, you will become more and more motivated to reach your goal.

We can't stress enough how crucial and important these first 3 weeks are to getting on track and forming this positive brain-expanding habit. You have taken this weekend to jump-start your challenge, which is a huge step toward achieving your goal. Once you get over the initial hump and into the groove, your new habit will be a piece of cake. Stay with it. Remember, this is something for your self-improvement, something you want for yourself, and something you deserve. You are on the road to being the person you want to be—your best you. We're so proud!

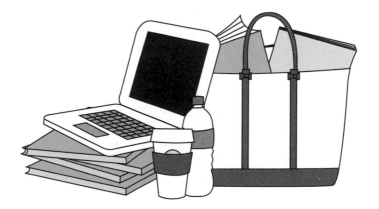

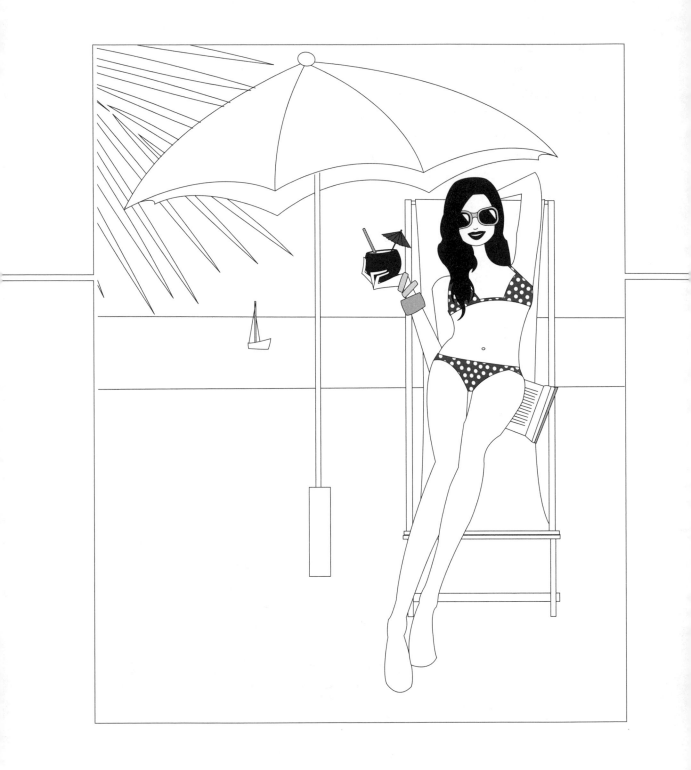

# Chapter Six
## Vacation Makeover

Aah, vacation. When was the last time you took one? This weekend makeover focuses on learning to create the time, budget, and know-how to help you take the extended holiday you've always dreamed of. Or maybe this weekend itself is the time off you desperately need right now!

It's truly amazing how much time goes by before we realize we haven't taken a break, gone on a trip, seen anyplace new, or even been out of our own environment in, well, maybe years. We know how busy you are, how expensive vacations can be, and how time just seems to escape. However, taking time off and getting away from everyday life is extremely important for mind, body, and soul. Depression and tension were nearly twice as high among rural women who took vacations only once in 2 years or once in 6 years compared with women who took vacations twice or more a year, according to a Wisconsin Rural Women's Health Study. Men at high risk for coronary heart disease who take advantage of their PTO (paid time off) days have a 39 percent lower risk of dying of heart disease, according to a study published in *Psychosomatic Medicine*.

## 10 INEXPENSIVE VACATION SPOTS

1. Destin, Florida
2. Huntington Beach, California
3. Las Vegas
4. Moab, Utah
5. Negril, Jamaica
6. Outer Banks, North Carolina
7. Placencia, Belize
8. Puerto Viejo, Costa Rica
9. San Francisco
10. Tulum, Mexico

We've asked you to take off this weekend as a mini-break, which might be more "vacation" than you've had in ages. Well, it seems an intervention was necessary. You need a break just to plan your break!

Here's what is great about a planned vacation: Not only is the vacation itself rejuvenating, spectacular, life changing, and [*insert your adjective of choice here!*], but the anticipation of the coming holiday is enough to elevate your mood, motivate you, and sustain you until the day you depart. The effect of vacation anticipation boosts happiness for 8 weeks, according to a study published in *Applied Research in Quality of Life*. And that holiday might be months away! Just knowing you have scheduled and can look forward to something rewarding and fabulous can change your state of mind.

Convinced yet?

# ☾ FRIDAY NIGHT

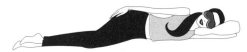

Where have you always wanted to go? You must have a list in your mind of all the places you fantasize about visiting. This list can (and probably will) contain locations both near and far, familiar and exotic. Perhaps there is a place you used to visit every summer as a child that you haven't been to in years and are dying to revisit. Or perhaps you're part of the 19 percent of newlyweds who never took that real honeymoon and have had a destination in mind ever since your engagement.

**Tonight, just dream.** Peruse travel magazines or surf the Internet. Go through those pages you tore out of travel sections over the years. Ask friends to suggest places they love. Write down your list of ideal vacation destinations and imagine yourself there.

## Jill

*I moved to Miami when I was 23 years old to be a sportscaster for CBS. It was a dream job. I covered the Miami Heat, Miami Dolphins, and Florida Marlins. Around that time, I met my first love. His name was David. We had an amazing young romance, and early on in the relationship we went with his family to Tahiti on a cruise. We visited five ports and spent 2 days bicycling around Bora-Bora looking for this special wholesale pearl lady. It was the happiest I had ever been. I dream about going back there one day with someone I am crazy about. This area is definitely high up on my list for an upcoming vacation. Although we were not meant to be, I still have the beautiful pearl necklace.*

## Dana

*I love to travel. However, there are still a million places I have never been and would love to see. These range from nearby places such as Savannah, Georgia (Gone with the Wind is one of my favorite books!), and New Orleans to destinations on the other side of the world such as the Seychelles (I am always searching for the ideal exotic beach locale). As much as I love to travel, I, too, need to make the effort to plan a vacation. Recently, I noticed that I hadn't been on a proper holiday in close to 5 years. My last big trip was to Australia. It took place when I was living in Miami, where I felt I was on constant holiday because my home was so close to the beach. Now that I am in New York, I still spend a ton of time in Miami, so it seems like I am on vacation a lot. But the reality is, I am always working when I am there, and my family is there, so Miami is never a completely relaxing time-out. When I finally realized this, I immediately planned and booked a yoga retreat to Tulum, Mexico. Within 3 weeks, I was on the plane. Anything is possible with a little research and planning!*

This weekend is your pre-escape escape. Have fun picturing yourself on holiday. You deserve to get away from your routine. This weekend gives you a bit of practice breaking out of your day-to-day habits—with the bonus, by Sunday night, of having planned an actual vacation to look forward to.

We know it can be uncomfortable to give yourself this time off, and it may take a bit of convincing yourself that you deserve to get away. The reality is you owe it to yourself. We can't stress enough how important a little R&R is. Believe us, your friends, family, and colleagues will appreciate your improved state of mind almost as much as you do!

You have set aside this weekend for this vacation-planning purpose. Enjoy the process of winding down, and relish your lack of commitment to anyone or anything besides yourself. This evening, when you make your list, don't worry about reality. We know money is a concern, time off is a concern, availability is a concern, kids versus no kids is a concern—the list goes on—but this process is supposed to be fun, not stressful. We'll tackle those issues tomorrow. Right now, fantasize. Go ahead. Try it.

This evening, have sweet dreams. We're sure you will. . . .

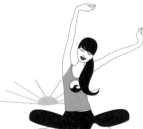

# SATURDAY MORNING

We hope you came up with an exciting fantasy list last night. Going forward, this list should be running and fluid, something you can reference every time you plan your next trip. (Yes, there will be a next trip after this one, and one after that.) As you travel, you can cross off the places you have visited; as you hear of new spots, you will add them to the list. Be careful: Taking a vacation can be habit forming!

This morning, get immersed in research to make your dream escape happen. As we mentioned, you probably have faraway fantasy destinations on your list as well as closer, more manageable getaways. We want you to experience all of them at some point, and with some smart saving and smart planning, you will!

However, we do want you to plan and take a vacation in the very near future, and we know that being realistic about your time, budget, and life is absolutely necessary. So we don't want you to quit your job and spend your life savings on that blowout trip around the world if that's not possible at the moment. Right now, the goal is to plan your first holiday. It can be short or long, close or far, economy or luxury. We're going to walk you through the process of finding the perfect time-out.

Some factors to consider when planning your holiday:

**Budget.** As with everything—clothing, restaurant meals, etc.—you can make less-expensive purchases and still get a rich experience. You can find a black purse at every price point, whether you are shopping on Rodeo Drive or at Target. You can have a lobster dinner at an exclusive restaurant or at a casual eatery. Either way, you will have had the experience of shopping and purchasing a handbag, and you will have had the experience of dining and eating a lobster. Maybe you will select the less-expensive restaurant so that you can splurge on the purse, or vice versa. It's all about picking and choosing when it comes to your budget and how you want to spend your money.

It's the same balancing act with travel. You can travel expensively or modestly or somewhere in between. If you have the time and the money, you can take a 2-week trip through Asia, or go on safari in South Africa, or jet around Europe. If that is not in the cards for you right now, at the very least, checking into a hotel in your own city for a night or two is an amazing way to get away from all your "stuff" at home and out of your day-to-day routine. And, of course, there is a middle ground, which can be anywhere from a long weekend to a weeklong excursion and be anything from a road trip to a plane ride away. Your destination can be in the States or a nearby country like Canada, Mexico, the Caribbean, or a distant locale like Hawaii (yes, we know that is a state!).

There are choices and compromises you can make to afford your dream destination. Maybe you fly coach class and splurge on the hotel, or maybe you don't splurge on either and are thrilled just to afford to reach your fantasy locale, or maybe you travel during the week instead of on the weekend so that the cost is lower. Regardless of how long you go away for, where you go, and how you get there, you experience time off and time away and come back to your daily life rested, replenished, and recharged, with some great memories to boot.

Several factors determine the cost of a trip. Asking the following questions will help you figure out how to make it work for your budget.

1. What is your ideal budget?
2. How much are plane tickets?
3. Do you have frequent-flier miles or points on a credit card?
4. Is driving an option?
5. Is the train an option?
6. Can you stay with friends or family or do you need a hotel or accommodations?
7. Do you need a rental car?
8. Is the trip all-inclusive or do activities and food cost extra?

Even if you are not in a position right now to afford your ultimate dream vacation, planning a less-expensive getaway not only allows you some time away; it also motivates you to make that fantasy vacation a reality. The trip planning could be as simple as setting up a "vacation account" at your bank and putting aside whatever you can afford every week or month, or out of every paycheck, however little (even $5, $10, or $20 at a time), to make sure you reach your goal!

**Dates.** We know you're busy with work, family, and other commitments that restrict the dates available for a vacation. Let's face it: There is always going to be *something* standing in the way of taking time off. The kids have school; you and/or your spouse have work; there are social commitments, holidays, and family obligations. You just need to make vacation as much of a priority. This is why you are planning now, so you can factor a holiday into your schedule with the least amount of disruption. To find the best dates, ask yourself these questions:

1. When would you ideally like to get away?

2. Are you bound by your kids' school vacations?

3. Is there a slower season at work?

4. Is it a big deal for you to miss a family holiday?

According to *The Complete Travel Detective Bible,* flying and booking your flight midweek will save you money. Airlines raise fares on Friday and lower them on Monday. Book your flight after the 7th of the month, since booking is busier right after paydays on the 1st and 15th.

**Time.** Sometimes you really need a break but can't afford to take 2 weeks off at one shot. Maybe you get only 2 weeks off per year and you'd rather divvy up the time. Or maybe work is just too crazy right now and you only have time to squeeze in a long weekend.

1. How much time can you afford to take off?

2. Are you looking to get away within the next couple of weeks or months?

3. Do you want to wait and plan a big trip for a few months out so everyone in your office knows in advance that your duties will need to be covered?

**Companions.** Who is this vacation for? Are you taking time off to recharge on your own, or are you traveling with your partner or a friend or a group of friends, or is it a family vacation? If it is just you, that will make the scheduling a lot easier and the transportation costs lower. Flying solo suits 11 percent of US adults, according to the US Travel Association. But solo travelers take slightly fewer vacations per year (4.3) than people who choose to travel with a friend (4.8). If you are going with a partner or friends, you will obviously need to find a time that works for both or all of you, but this trip could be more cost effective, as the per-person rate will be lower if you share accommodations. If you are traveling as a family, the cost of flights, food, etc., will rise, but you may be able to get great family packages that make the trip affordable.

1. How many plane or train tickets do you need?

2. Will you be sharing a room?

3. Can you get a group or family rate?

4. Will you be traveling during a school holiday or the summer?

5. If you are going with your spouse only, do you need a sitter for the kids, or can they stay with your parents or friends?

**Destination.** Which came first, the chicken or the egg? The location of your ideal getaway can determine how much time off you need, when you can go, and how much the trip will cost—or vice versa. If none of those factors are an issue, just pick a spot, book it, and enjoy!

Going someplace farther away—out of the country, for example—will ideally be a longer trip and will likely cost more than a weekend getaway within driving distance. If you can't afford the time or the expense right now, perhaps something local will suit your needs.

1. Where is your ideal vacation getaway?

2. How long will it take to get there (travel time)?

3. Is this place seasonal—summer or winter?

4. Is it dependent on weather—sun or snow?

5. Do you need expensive equipment—skis, golf clubs?

Lots to consider, huh? We know it can seem overwhelming. But here's the plus side: Once the logistical stuff is handled and planned, the holiday is pure enjoyment from there on out, from the excitement and anticipation right through to the relaxation and fun. The priceless benefits of a getaway range from stress reduction to memories that last a lifetime. It's totally worth it and totally addicting.

With a bit of organization, planning a trip isn't difficult. These days, you can pretty much book everything online. When you sit down this morning to start looking at your options, you'll realize that trip planning is primarily a matter of booking flights and/or accommodations. Once you've picked your destination and your transportation and lodging are sorted, you're home free to design the rest of your trip at leisure.

**Prioritize.** Determine which factor is highest on your priority list—time, budget, or destination—and what is most flexible. Start there. Either pick the dates and the amount of time you can get away; or decide how much you are willing to spend; or determine that no matter what, you are determined to go to Mexico, Japan, or Nashville!

Maybe right now you have only the time or the budget for a long weekend jaunt within driving distance. Or maybe you have time for that trip to the other side of the world—the honeymoon you never took—before you start your new job. If time is your priority, decide how much time and when, and put those dates in the calendar.

Once you have selected your dates, figure out where you can realistically and affordably go in that time frame. Work down your priority list. Which is the next biggest priority—budget or locale? With that information in hand, start searching for flights and accommodations.

Perhaps money is tight and you want to get away, but the really fabulous vacation will have to wait. Or perhaps you can afford a first-class vacation, but you've just been too lazy to plan it. Either way, calculate how much you are comfortable spending.

Once you have your budget, again work down your priority list. Perhaps your dates are flexible, but you really want to go to Spain, or California, or Fiji. Or perhaps you are less concerned with where you go and more eager to take advantage of a certain window to get away. Decide that and start looking at some options for your destination choice and your availability.

If the destination is your priority and your dates and budget are flexible, start checking your options. For a seasonal location, like a winter hot spot in the Caribbean or Mexico or Florida, the rates will be lower in the summertime. You'll still get the same relaxing beach holiday. Temperatures may be a bit hotter, but hey, you're on the beach anyway, with a beautiful ocean, and you might be lucky enough to avoid the crowds! If someplace like Europe is your dream destination, but it's a bit pricey during the summer high season, try booking between late fall and spring for a better deal and fewer tourists.

Some other things to keep in mind when you are planning your getaway:

**Discount travel Web sites.** The Internet offers a wealth of information, and there are great deals to be had. Sites like Kayak.com, Expedia.com, and Priceline.com are great places to start. They offer deals on flights, hotels, and rental cars. Individual airlines' Web sites are easy to navigate and have great prices if you are flexible on time of day and day of travel. But be wary of deals that sound too good to be true—do your research so you know a good deal when you see it and can avoid scams. Fridays and Sundays are usually the busiest and most expensive travel days, because everyone is scheduling around the weekend and not missing work. If you can avoid those travel days, you will get better rates.

**Frequent-flier miles or credit card points.** If you have either of these, you can save yourself a lot of money. These can be used for flights and/or hotels and even a rental car at your destination, if you need one. It's worth looking into your options using miles or points. Sometimes it seems we just collect and save these and never use them! Miles and points can be especially handy if you wish to travel sooner rather than later, as rates are generally higher the closer to your travel date. You still might be able to afford your trip if you have frequent-flier options in your arsenal. Also, if your travel plans change, tickets booked with miles are generally changeable, whereas most airlines will charge a change fee to reschedule a regular ticket.

*Consumer Reports* magazine offers insight on what to look for when comparing cards. At this writing, Chase Sapphire offers 25,000 points—promoted as worth $250 toward a round-trip flight—after you spend $3,000 in the first 3 months. American Express offers a "preferred" version of its Blue Sky and Blue Cash cards—both with a $75 annual fee, but you get a $100 sign-up bonus and better cash-back options than the no-annual-fee versions. Want to avoid an annual fee? You can still rack up the miles. The no-fee Capital One Venture One Rewards card offers 1.25 miles per $1 spent. If choosing an airline's card, look for

*Jill* *I love frequent-flier miles. I love that when I buy something at Saks, I can rationalize it because I get miles on my American Express card with every dollar I spend! Just the other day, my girlfriend invited me to go to Greece. She goes with her family for a month every summer, and she asked me to join them in Mykonos. On 1 week's notice, I booked an airline flight (that would otherwise have cost a fortune) using frequent-flier miles. I can't wait. I just hit my favorite boutiques to get a few must-haves for my trip. (The charges will go toward my next adventure, of course!)*

*Dana* *Several years ago, a friend of mine was going to travel around Spain alone, trip already booked. I decided to join at the last minute (literally 10 days out). I went online and found a great deal on Expedia.com for an airline ticket round-trip from LAX to Madrid. Within 5 minutes, I had booked my trip. Within 2 weeks, I was on holiday. It can be that easy and that affordable!*

special perks, such as travel insurance, trip-delay coverage, rental-car insurance, and no foreign transaction fees.

**Advance booking.** Generally, the farther in advance you book your airline ticket, the better the ticket price, especially if you wish to travel during busy peak holiday times. Most airlines rates go up if the flight is within 1 week's time, so if you can book at least 7 days in advance, you will have a better rate than if you reserved at the last minute. The exceptions are last-minute deals offered by airlines to fill seats on certain flights—obviously useful only if your travel schedule is extremely flexible.

**Packages.** If you are flying and staying in a hotel, often you can get a package deal that will bring the overall trip price down. Sometimes transportation to and from the airport and hotel will be included. Packages are definitely worth investigating if you know you need both services.

**All-inclusive resorts/cruises/tours.** If you are looking for a getaway where you don't even have to figure out where to eat dinner, an all-inclusive option might be perfect for you. Not only are the rates usually better on these types of trips, but all the excursions, meals, and activities are already organized and planned. You can either participate or not, depending on what you feel like on any given day.

**Adventure.** If you prefer to be left to your own devices to explore and get immersed in local culture, you may simply want to secure a place to stay and a flight, train, or car to get to your destination. Since flights are expensive to change, make sure you have reserved a place to stay before you pay for the flight. That way you can change the room dates if there are no flights available on the days you select or if the flights are less expensive a day or so before or after the dates you initially chose.

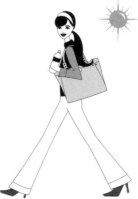

# SATURDAY AFTERNOON

Take a little break, have a relaxing lunch, and think about your options. You did a great job researching and narrowing them down. Your vacation is within sight.

**Reserve it.** Once you have figured out where you are going, when you are going, with whom you are going, and have found transportation and lodging in your budget, it's time to book that trip!

Double-check your calendar for conflicts, then put the dates down for your trip. Confer with any travel companions to make sure you are on the same page with all the arrangements, dates, costs, etc. Commit to the plan together. If you are staying with family or friends at your destination, confirm the dates with them.

Most hotels have a 48-hour cancellation policy, so reserving rooms is usually no problem. Car rental agencies don't charge you until you pick up the car, so you should be fine in that department, too. If the airline allows it, put the flights on hold for 24 hours. If the airline doesn't allow you to hold a reservation, or you are booking on one of the discount sites, and you are 100 percent sure you can take the time off, can afford the trip, and are excited about the destination, then go for it and book the trip! Either way, you will be booked by tomorrow, so it's just a matter of whether you take the plunge now or in the morning. Yes, you are really doing this! You deserve it.

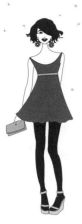

## SATURDAY NIGHT

If your vacation destination has a culture, cuisine, and language different from your own, gear yourself up for the trip by having that country's cuisine for dinner. You can cook for yourself, if that is something you enjoy. Or celebrate your impending vacation at a restaurant—Mexican, Chinese, Japanese, Italian, French, or whatever relates to your trip.

After dinner, put together a few travel outfits. Going to the Bahamas? Dig out those fun beach dresses. Hiking in the Andes? Pull out your trail boots. Get into the vibe and the culture. Try to wrap your head around the idea that you will be experiencing the real thing sooner than you know!

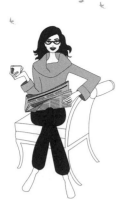

## SUNDAY

Follow up on any pending questions or details that you worked through yesterday. Once you've resolved loose ends and are in the free and clear to commit, book your trip.

Congrats! You are on your way. You may not realize it until you get back from your adventure (although we think trip anticipation is just as exciting and rewarding as the event itself), but your entire mood will change for the better. You'll feel relaxed, rejuvenated, and ready to take on the rest of your regular life. Experiencing a vacation is wonderful and necessary for your mental health—and that better frame of mind benefits everyone around you, too.

Make a list of people who need to be aware of your absence—boss, co-workers, family, etc. Plan to notify them on Monday morning. By setting this trip in stone, you'll feel confident about taking the time off and allow yourself to feel excited!

**Start packing!** Now that the trip is booked, today you celebrate and get ready for your upcoming vacation. It doesn't matter if your trip is next week or next month. This is your weekend to make over your vacation life. That means shopping! What's more fun than getting gear for your trip?

In fact, nothing gets you in the mood to travel more than shopping for something new to wear or use while you are away. If you are hitting the beach, maybe it's a new bikini, hat, sandals, caftan, sunglasses, or good book to read. If you are checking out a new city for the first time, a guidebook of museums, restaurants, shops, etc., is a great purchase, as are comfortable yet fashionable walking shoes or a cute dress for a night out on the town. If your trip is athletic, perhaps you want to splurge on new equipment—golf clubs or skis? No matter where you are going, the right luggage, a camera, and an iPod are key items.

If you're traveling out of the country, make sure your passport is current. If you booked a trip last minute and need to rush your passport, be prepared to pay additional fees plus overnight delivery costs. If you're renewing, check online to see if you qualify to renew by mail—and determine what forms you'll need to fill out to do so. It's a good idea to decide in advance how much money you'll want to spend on your trip and if you will use a credit card, prepaid debit card, or traveler's checks. Be smart about money and valuables. Don't take anything of great value like expensive or sentimental jewelry.

This is your first vacation of many to come. Yes, we know it's easy to get into a routine and rut, to say that you'll plan something when you have the time but then never make the time to make the time. Not only are 20 percent of us chronic procrastinators, according to a 1996 study in *Psychological Reports*, but also 57 percent of employees who receive paid time off don't use all of their allotted time, says a survey by Harris Interactive. Well, you have now planned to take the time. You are going to have a fabulous holiday in the near future.

Remember, this is not a one-time deal. Now that you know how easy it can be

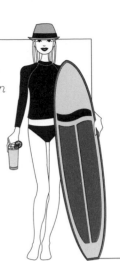

*Jill* I have a strict packing rule. Unless I am going away for more than a week, I don't bring more than a carry-on. (Obviously, this excludes a vacation where I need equipment, like skis.) I like to keep it simple. More choices lead to more confusion. I pack only my favorite things, which can be mixed and matched, and this leaves me with fewer choices and less stress. It works. Trust me.

*Dana* My ideal holiday is usually on a beach, so even when I don't have a trip planned, I am collecting things that I will eventually use. I have more bathing suits than I care to disclose. Sarongs and flip-flops, too. I have the perfect wheelie luggage that fits in the overhead bin, because I hate to check luggage no matter how far or for how long I travel. I never leave home without my iPod, even if I am just going to the market. I generally don't take any jewelry other than what I am wearing and know I won't take off. And I never get on a plane without my passport, even if I am flying within the States. I am of the mind-set that a great travel opportunity could come up at any time, even if I'm already out of town, and I always want to be prepared!

to plan, and how much fun it is to have something to look forward to, make a pact with yourself that you will continue to map out future vacations. The best thing you can do to never fall back into the no-vacation rut is to schedule your next trip as soon as you return from this one. As long as you have something on the horizon, your mood will improve, you'll find it easier to get through tough days, and you'll notice an overall lightness in your step. We're not making this up. It is a real thing. We're so excited for you! Can we come?

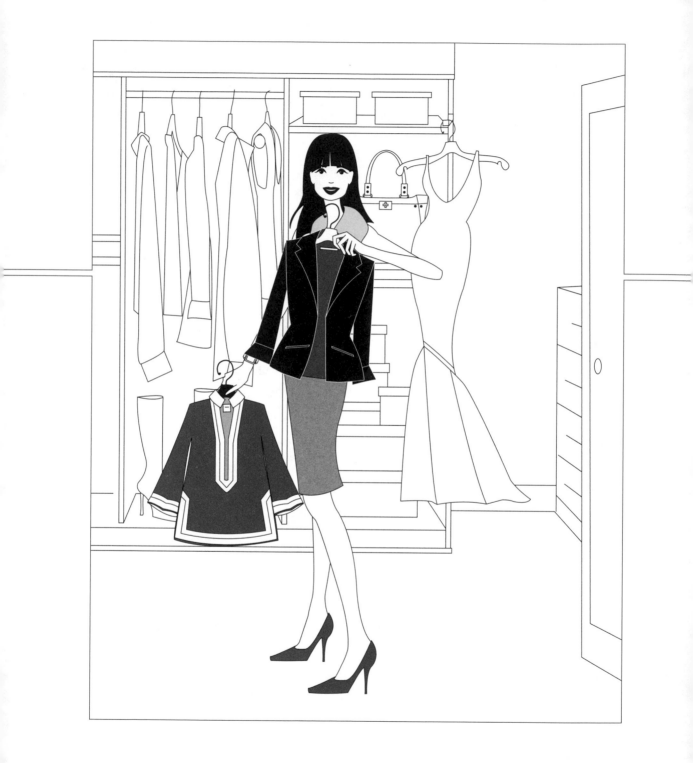

# *Chapter Seven*
# Closet Makeover

If you thought you found a ton of stuff that you didn't need (or that didn't belong) in your fridge in Chapter 1 or in your makeup vanity in Chapter 3, just wait until you get to your closet! Yes, it's likely that your closet is a vast wasteland of neglected, ill-fitting items that are also in, how shall we say, not such great condition. Are we close?

Do you hold on to suits from a job you no longer have? Do those suits feature 1980s shoulder pads? Or maybe you have maternity clothes that don't fit and you won't need again. What about the garments that sport their original price tags—even though they are not recent purchases? Only 6 percent of women surveyed in a Talbots National Fit Study said they wear all their clothes on a regular basis. But when people took the time to clean out their closet, they not only saved time and felt calmer; they also had more productive shopping experiences because they knew what they already owned and what they really liked.

Sound familiar? We thought it might. Well, this weekend we are going to remedy that closet chaos. By Sunday evening, you will have a cleaned-out, organized, and fully functioning closet with all the items you do need and none of the items you don't.

Are you ready to get down and dirty and make hard-core decisions about what will stay and what will depart from your wardrobe? This is your weekend to dedicate to this project. We promise you are going to feel (and ultimately look) like a new person by the time you're through.

## ☾ FRIDAY NIGHT

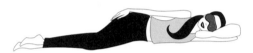 Cleaning out and organizing your closet is a big project, so tonight we just want you to mentally prepare yourself for the weekend (and get some garbage bags ready!). You are going to get rid of a bunch of stuff that no longer serves your purposes and is causing unnecessary clutter and confusion. If you'd like to have a friend help you through this, we're all for a little emotional support. Choose someone you know will be honest, someone you are completely comfortable with. There are going to be a lot of wardrobe try-ons and tough decisions ahead.

Here's the goal of this weekend: Every remaining item in your closet must be considered a "10"—meaning on a scale of 1 to 10, it is the best. And each must receive yes answers to the following criteria questions to remain in your wardrobe:

1. Is the garment in perfect condition—no holes, no pills, and no stains?
2. Does it represent your personality—meaning do you feel like *you* when you wear it?
3. Does it fit your lifestyle—meaning do you have occasion to wear it?
4. Is it age appropriate?
5. Is it location/climate appropriate?
6. Do you wear or have you ever actually worn it?

_Jill_ Once a week (still), I get a call from my mother saying, "I got rid of all the 9s." My mother (as I've mentioned before) keeps everything, and she, like many people, finds it hard to part with things. The way I got her to purge is that we made a deal: When she rids herself of anything that is not a 10, she earns credit toward shopping for new pieces. We have a one-in, five-out rule! For every five items she dismisses from her closet, she is allowed to buy one new. We like our little process. You can adapt it accordingly. I only have items in my closet that fit me perfectly and are comfortable and that I wouldn't have a problem running into my ex-boyfriend in. Even when I am in my sweats, I feel fabulous.

_Dana_ A long time ago, I made a promise to myself that I would no longer wear or buy anything that wasn't a 10. The difference between wearing something that makes you feel confident, sexy, and totally you and throwing on something that is just okay (because you are only running out for a coffee and the paper) is huge. I realized I always exercise the option to wear the cute, flattering outfit if I don't own anything that is not cute. I learned this lesson quickly the first time I ran into my ex in a not-so-cute outfit, and I won't ever let that happen again!

7. Does it fit in with your personal style?

8. Does it fit and flatter your figure perfectly?

You will ask these eight questions about each and every piece of clothing—but not until the morning. This evening, relax, have a healthy dinner, and get to bed early so you can start in the morning with a fresh, clear mind and a rested body.

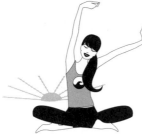

# SATURDAY MORNING

Are you ready to get started? If you have recruited a trusted friend for help, tell her (or him!) to come on over. While this is a big project, we hope you see it as a fun activity. You should definitely have a lot of laughs—especially the first time you do a massive cleanout. Get a little nourishment in your stomach to sustain you. Let's get started!

You will go through your closet and inspect and try on each item one by one. And, yes, this does include shoes, handbags, and accessories as well as under-garments and sleepwear. As you go, you will place each item on one of five piles:

✓ *Keep.* Anything that is a perfect 10, meaning in perfect condition, in keeping with your style, representing your personality, age appropriate, lifestyle appropriate, fits and flatters your frame and makes you look and feel sexy and beautiful—and, of course, something you actually do wear.

*Consign.* Anything that is current or vintage that has a designer label.

✓ *Donate.* Anything that is in decent condition but doesn't have financial value.

*Toss.* Anything that is not in good condition, meaning not saleable or wearable.

*Maybe.* This is where the consign/donate/toss items make a pit stop on their way to their proper and respective piles. (We know sometimes it's hard to choose!)

Where you place an item depends on how you answered the criteria questions on pages 108–9. Let's look at these criteria more closely.

**Condition.** First, if the garment is not in perfect condition, it has no place in your closet, and there is no need for you to try it on. If it is ripped, stained, stretched out, pilly (with the little nubs that form on sweaters and knits), yellowed, or full of holes, it can go straight into the toss or donate pile. You will have to make the judgment call here as to what shape it is in: whether it is worth donating or can be simply tossed in the trash.

**Personality.** If the item passed the condition test and is still in the game, the next question to ask is whether or not it represents your personality. When you go into your closet to pick out an outfit, is this garment something you feel totally comfortable in? Does it make you feel good?

Do you have a big personality and wear clothing that is bright or patterned, or do you have a reserved personality and feel more comfortable in solids and neutrals? In most cases, even if you bought something and felt excited about it at the time, if it's been sitting in your closet for a while, or if when you wore it you didn't feel that great, it's not 100 percent *you*—and you know where it goes! Out! Decide if it is a great piece that you can sell to earn a little money back at the consignment shop or if it is something you will just donate.

**Lifestyle.** Next, ask if this garment fits into your lifestyle. Over the years, we go through many shifts in our day-to-day environment. Some people change jobs or careers, others choose motherhood as their path and move out of the corporate or work environment. Here are some general closet essentials, depending on your lifestyle.

## WARDROBE ESSENTIALS FOR EVERY WOMAN

### Corporate

Chic suit

Fitted blouse

Black pumps

Structured day bag

Conservative jewelry—watch, stud earrings

### Creative

Fashion-forward dress/skirt

Feminine blouse

Strappy sandals

Edgy purse

Statement earrings or necklace

*Casual*

Dark denim jeans

Fitted T-shirt/tank/sweater

Ballet flats

Oversize day bag

Simple jewelry—necklace with small charms

Every time you make a big lifestyle change, your wardrobe likely needs to change, too. So even if the clothes still look like you, they don't really *act* like you. If they are in good condition and still fit, the usual rationale is, "Why get rid of them?" Well, if the clothes don't fit in your life anymore, the reason is because you don't need them and they are taking up valuable space! If these clothes are office appropriate, they can go to good use for women who need work clothes and can't afford them. Great charities such as Dress for Success will place your unnecessary but useful pieces into the right hands.

**Age appropriateness.** Not only does our occupation change over time; so does our age. There's nothing worse than someone trying to look younger by wearing clothing designed for a woman 20 years her junior. For that matter, if you are on the younger side, the last thing you need to be doing is wearing clothing that is too matronly or aging. This discrepancy tends to be more obvious in trendier items rather than classic pieces.

The guideline as you age is to keep the hemline a little longer, the colors a bit more muted, the patterns a little less wild, and the accessories tamer. If you enjoy participating in the latest trends, by all means do, just use this guideline to keep your selections age appropriate. As you continue to go through your closet, bear this rule in mind and make sure each garment finds its way into the appropriate pile.

**Location/climate appropriateness.** Another thing that may change once, twice, or several times in our lives is where we live. Some people move from the big city to the suburbs or the country, or vice versa. Others move from a warm climate to a cold one, or vice versa. With these changes, your wardrobe needs to change as well—otherwise you end up in the situation of saving, storing, or hoarding items you no longer use.

Ask yourself if you really need those heavy sweaters you wore in Vermont now that you live in Florida, or if you really need those fancy shoes and dresses that you wore in New York City but have never once put on now that you live in Idaho. Be honest. We know how hard it is to part with anything that is still in good condition and that you once loved and lived in, but if you don't wear it anymore, it's really of no use to you—and it might be useful to someone else.

**Telltale tags.** Do any of your items still carry price tags? We know how cute the garment was in the magazine or on the mannequin, and you just *had* to have it, but once you got it home, it wasn't *you*. Right? The honest truth is, if you haven't worn it yet, you are not going to. (Obviously, if it is very recently purchased, we can't make that call, but we are talking about the items that have been sitting for months, years even, with the tags still on.) These have got to go, now.

Because the item is brand-new (or relatively new), depending on how current or still in fashion it is or whether it has a designer label, you may be able to recoup some of your money if you sell the garment on consignment. Or you can donate the barely worn to Goodwill or another charity. Either way, clearing out "tagged" items relieves you of the guilt that comes from buying clothes and never wearing them. Whether you have a little extra cash in hand or have made a clothing donation, you'll feel warm and fuzzy inside. Pick your pile accordingly!

If the garment doesn't have a price tag, but you haven't worn it in years, chances are very good that you will never wear it again. Once something falls out of rotation, it pretty much enters the black hole known as the dark recesses of your closet, never to be seen or worn again. Thus, if it is in decent condition, into the consignment or donation pile it goes. According to the company California Closets, people tend to stop wearing a certain item after 6 months. Here's the company's tip for getting equal use out of all of your clothes: "Place hangers in backward and return items to the closet with the hanger facing forward. After six months, remove clothing that has not been worn [the 'backward hangers'] and store elsewhere or give to charity."

**Personal style.** This is another important consideration when deciding whether or not an item should stay in your wardrobe. When we talk about personal style, we mean your "look," your "uniform"—your go-to outfit. Of course, what you wear to brunch will not be the same as what you wear for an evening out on the town, but what we mean is your "vibe."

Personal style is about dressing as an extension of your personality. Most people will fall into one of the following style categories:

*Classic.* She mostly wears classic basics in neutral colors. Think dark denim jeans, a white button-down top, ballet flats, and an Hermès Kelly-type bag.

*Bohemian.* The bohemian wears flowy, feminine tops and dresses. Think embroidered tunic top, white jeans, gold open-toe sandals, and a hobo bag.

*Sporty.* Athletic wear or athletically inspired is this person's clothing of choice. Think long-sleeve T-shirt and short shorts over a bikini and Ugg Australia boots.

*Preppie.* Think country club garb: polo shirts and cable knit sweaters in pinks, greens, white, and navy.

*Fashionista.* She is always on trend and usually a little fancy, too. Mostly in black, and always in high heels. Think sophisticated and put-together.

*Casual chic.* Easy and comfortable, but always cute. Most moms fall into this category. Think T-shirts and jeans and cute sneaks or post-yoga/Pilates gear.

You will likely fall into one of the above style categories, or a combination of two. When you find your style and stick with it, all your clothing is effortlessly mix-and-matchable. It's when you get swayed by all the latest trends and start buying clothing from all the different styles that your look can get befuddled. This makes it a problem to figure out what to wear. It will slow you down every day when you are trying to get dressed and will have your closet cluttered and a bit overwhelming. Sorting this out during your closet cleanout is a must.

Be honest with yourself about who you are and what your style is. Make peace with letting the other items go. Again, if these garments are in good condition, but just aren't *you,* find a pile that will lead them to their proper home.

**Flattering fit.** Last, whatever has made the cut and is still in your keep pile must be tried on now. Yes, every single item. This is the only way you will know if the item fits you properly and flatters your figure. Obviously, those that don't fit should be donated or consigned or, if possible, tailored to fit you. Hemming too-long pants and taking in a jacket are simple alterations that will make ordinary pieces fit you perfectly so you look and feel your best—plus, they'll remain integral pieces in your wardrobe repertoire.

Be very clear here about what is truly a 10 and what is not. Does the garment make you feel fantastic, confident, and as though you could take on the world? Or

*Jill*
*I am a classic girl at heart, but, oh, do I love my accessories. Whenever you see me off duty, I will likely be in jeans and a T-shirt and flip-flops or ballet flats, but I will always have on some sort of fabulous statement piece of jewelry. I don't think there is any better way to have fun with fashion than with a statement necklace or earrings or a big cocktail ring. It makes even the most basic outfit pop, and it brings out the fashionista in me!*

*Dana*
*My style is definitely bohemian with a little fashionista thrown in. I live in pretty, feminine tops, jeans, and dresses, and I also enjoy experimenting with the trends when they work with my style. My favorite stores are Calypso St. Barth and Tomas Maier, and my go-to dress is always from Michelle Jonas. I have learned that even though I can appreciate the other styles, I don't end up wearing those pieces, so I no longer have them in my wardrobe. This saves me a lot of time, money, and confusion, not to mention unnecessary clutter!*

is it sorta dumpy and you're just keeping it to run down the street for coffee or to do laundry? Well, there is no sorta dumpy allowed here. If you don't feel like a million bucks in it, toss it! Think of it this way: If you were out running errands in this outfit, and a friend called with an impromptu invite to lunch, would you feel cute enough to go without running home to change first? We're not talking black tie, just dressing well for simple occasions.

If you have a trusted friend helping you today, listen to her or his opinion carefully. You don't want anything back in your closet that shouldn't be there. This includes shoes, handbags, and all accessories, too. If the shoe is uncomfortable or not exactly the right size, it is not exactly yours anymore. Got it?

**Wear me maybe?** Hopefully, most pieces ended up in the keep, donate, consign, or toss piles. But we know that some pieces slipped through the cracks and ended up in your maybe pile. Really, truthfully, honestly look at those items again. Trust your first instinct, which was that they aren't an automatic keep. Yes, that means that those items probably should be donated, sold, or tossed. If you were lukewarm about them during the first round, you definitely won't miss them. We promise.

What a productive morning. Good job! Are you starting to feel lighter already? Take a little break, have a nice lunch, but don't go too far. We have more to do this afternoon.

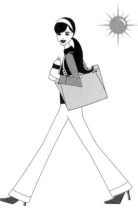

# SATURDAY AFTERNOON

Now we are going to deal with all the clothes you are not keeping. By the end of this afternoon, those clothes that are not part of your perfect-10 wardrobe will be out of the house, so that by tomorrow evening you will have a clutter-free, functional closet.

Whatever is in the toss pile (items that are unsalvage-able) can now be thrown out. Stained, torn, stretched out, something that no one should be wearing—you get the idea.

*Jill* With our last book, I Have Nothing to Wear!, we had women in a frenzy. Dana and I toured around the country urging women to get rid of 75 percent of what was in their closets. Mouths dropped, gasps were heard around the room, and one woman shouted, "Yeah, right!" after we made that statement. Once everyone went home and starting sorting through their closets, they realized how right we were. We think you should always look and feel your best when you go to work, go to the gym, or run to get a cup of coffee. The reality is, we all have too much to wear. I had a pair of Missoni pants that I bought at T.J. Maxx for 75 percent off plus another 20 percent discount. They were designer, and they were perfect, but there was one problem—they did not look perfect on me. They are now at the consignment shop. Now I have room for a new piece that does look fabulous!

*Dana* I have been cleaning out my closet for years, so I don't need a major closet overhaul anymore. However, I do a serious cleanout twice a year—usually spring and fall. I take stock of everything and decide what stays and what goes. In the interim, I am constantly retiring and donating, consigning, or tossing pieces that should not be there. One of my favorite errands is to drop off my "donate" and "consign" items at the appropriate spot. There is a Salvation Army only 3 blocks from my apartment, so even if it's just a couple of things, I'd rather drop them off at the consignment shop or donation center than have them in my closet!

Take the consignment items to the appropriate shop near you. You might need to do a little research to locate a shop. TheThriftShopper.Com and NARTS: The Association of Resale Professionals (www.narts.org) offer great search engines. If the pieces are high-end designer and/or vintage, there are consignment shops that cater to this market. If the garments or accessories are not high-end but have recognizable labels, there are resale shops that cater to this level of merchandise as well. And if you have the time and are really up for a project (for another day), there is always eBay! Or this fabulous new site Poshmark.com. Poshmark is like Instagram only you use it to buy and sell clothes. Just snap a pic of the item with your phone and post. It's that easy!

Next, take the donation items to a nearby donation center or favorite charity. If you have work clothes in your donate pile, you might offer these to Dress for Success (find locations at www.dressforsuccess.org), then give the rest to either Goodwill, the Salvation Army, or a battered women's shelter. Your gifts are always so appreciated.

You must feel great by now. The purging alone is cathartic—that same California Closets survey found that 43 percent of women feel relaxed and in control with better organization. And knowing that you are helping other women in need is also rewarding. Just wait till you make a little money from your consigned items and get a little tax break from your donations!

The first part of your mission is accomplished, but you still have a pile of stuff you are keeping and an empty closet. We remedy that next. To get your closet in the best shape possible, you need a few organizational supplies.

Let's hit the stores. Target, the Container Store, or Bed Bath & Beyond should have everything on this list.

**Felt hangers.** These will quadruple your hanging space because they are so thin, and the felt grips your clothes so that nothing falls off—even your spaghetti-strap tops and dresses will cling to the hanger without sliding. The added bonus is that they make your closet aesthetically pleasing: Having uniform hangers is so much prettier than all those random plastic, wood, and dry-cleaning hangers you were using.

**Plastic shoe and boot boxes.** These see-through, stackable storage boxes give each pair of shoes and boots a happy home and make it so easy to see your shoe choices when you look in the closet. These, too, will make your closet prettier and more organized. No more piles of shoes that force you to search for the mate to the pair that you want to wear.

**Hanging jewelry organizer.** This canvas contraption with plastic see-through pouches provides each pair of earrings, necklace, bracelet, and ring with its own little compartment. No more tangled or mangled jewelry, and no missing earring to the pair. The organizer takes up minimal space because it hangs thinly in your closet, and its clear pouches save you a ton of time when looking for that perfect accessory.

**Hanging purse organizer.** This is a canvas storage piece for your bags, if you don't have any other space for them. It provides a little shelf for each purse with easy access for you to see and reach the right bag for your outfit.

If you found any other great organizational items at the store that you think you can use, grab those, too.

## ADDITIONAL USEFUL ORGANIZATIONAL ITEMS

Belt hanger

Drawer organizers (for jewelry/socks/underwear/scarves)

Drawer/shelf liners

Hat boxes

Shelf dividers

Stackable drawers

You've had a busy and successful day so far. We don't want you to overdo it. We know this weekend is for you, and even though it's about getting your closet in tip-top shape, we want you to enjoy it. When you get home, put your new supplies near the closet and organize your "keep" pile out of the way as well. You

*Jill* *I believe everyone should have a closet that looks as organized and as pretty as Carrie Bradshaw's from* Sex and the City. *Even if you have a tiny space, you can still make it look spectacular. Believe me, I have lived in the smallest apartments with the littlest closets, but the one thing I always do is make my setup functional and fashionable. So, of course, I decided to create my own line of items that will whip any closet into shape in seconds (all available at QVC.com). Haute Hangers (thin felt hangers) and Mini-Mannequins (to display jewelry) are two of my favorite products. Since I am constantly accessorizing, I like to have all of my jewelry in full view. I set this little mannequin right on my vanity, and my jewelry is displayed as though it were art. I no longer have a ball of tangled chains lying in my drawer, my jewelry is organized (necklaces in front, earrings in back), and my bedroom looks like a boutique!*

*Dana* *About 2 years ago, I switched my closet over to felt hangers. I don't know how to describe the feeling I get every time I open the doors—still to this day. It literally makes me smile to see everything hanging so prettily and organized. I have always saved shoeboxes, and I store all of my shoes and boots in their respective boxes, which keeps them stacked, paired, and organized. But I think I may take it to the next level and switch them all over to the clear boxes!*

are going to tackle your closet organization next, and by the end of tomorrow you will be sorted, but for today you've done enough!

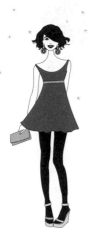

# SATURDAY NIGHT

Reward yourself tonight with a healthy, satisfying dinner or a relaxing bath or both. If you had a partner or friend helping you today with your closet cleanout, treat him or her to dinner to say thanks and have a laugh about all the ridiculous things you tried on today! Offer to return the favor, because we're sure your partner or friend has items that are laughable, too!

Have some fun and experiment with new looks from your "keep" pile to wear out this evening. We know it's not all organized and hanging in your closet beautifully yet, but take a look at what's in there. We bet there are pieces you didn't even know you had.

Now that you have a better idea of your style and know that all the items work together:

- Mix and match some new pairings.

- Throw on a dress instead of the same old jeans that you (used to) store so conveniently on the chair in your bedroom.

- Be bold with accessories. Break out that necklace you love but never wear, or the fabulous earrings or ring. Get out of your jewelry rut.

- Now that you've found the missing shoe to your favorite pair, rejoice and kick up your heels. The cleanout was worth this alone!

- Pare down to a clutch—no need to tote your huge day bag that has everything you need and tons of stuff you don't.

Take it up a notch. Celebrate your new closet, wardrobe, and the perfect "10" that is you.

Then get a good night's sleep. You have more real work to do in the morning. Sleep well. . . .

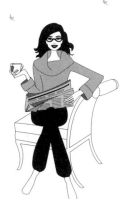

# SUNDAY

Good morning! Make sure you have a nourishing breakfast, because today we are going into the trenches of your closet. You'll need focus, energy, and stamina.

At this point, everything should be out of your closet. You are starting fresh, as though you are moving into a new place. If you have built-ins and your closet is gorgeous even when empty, lucky you. If not, with the aid of your organizational supplies, you will ultimately have a beautiful closet, too. Either way, the following guidelines will help you reach your goal.

**Hang it like art.** Break out your felt hangers and begin with your hanging items: dresses, blouses, skirts, pants (jeans can be folded or hung, depending on your preference and how much room you have), and blazers. Organize these by type of garment and color. Working from left to right, hang long dresses together, short dresses, blouses and tops, short skirts, long skirts, pants (and jeans), and, last, blazers. Within these categories, group items by color from dark to light, or vice versa.

Organizing this way provides space in the center of your closet underneath the shorter items. This is where you stack your shoe boxes so you can see them (we'll talk more about this in a moment). The organization also makes it much easier to pull together an outfit. If you are in the mood for a long dress, they will be grouped together. If you are looking for a skirt or pants/jeans and a blouse, these will be grouped next to one another so you can easily see your combination choices without having to weed through dresses, too. Finally, you can polish off your outfit with a blazer from the end of the row. Organizing by color also makes it easier to find things and shows you how many of each item you own in the same hue and lets you decide if you really need or wear all of them or if any are duplicates you can toss.

**Stack the shelves.** Next, on your shelf or shelves, neatly fold and stack the following: sweaters, sweats, T-shirts, tank tops, workout clothes, sleepwear, and any knit items that should not be hung (knits stretch when stored on a hanger, so even knit dresses should be folded). Keep these organized first according to category and then by color (light to dark, or vice versa) within each category. If you chose not to hang your jeans, they can be folded and placed on the shelf. Make sure everything is visible and your piles are neat.

**Store the shoes.** Take the shoes and boots you are keeping and give each pair its own special box. You will be amazed how nice this looks and how manageable it will be when you are rushing and looking for the right shoe to polish off your outfit. Stack the boots together and then make separate stacks each for closed-toe flats, closed-toe pumps, open-toe heels, and open-toe flat sandals. Place these boxes on the closet floor underneath the shorter dresses, skirts, and blouses so that you can see what's in each box and none of your longer dresses or pants get crushed. If you are really pressed for space, there is always the option of storing your shoe boxes underneath the bed, where they can be easily reached.

**Organize bags.** If you don't have spare shelf space for your handbags and purses, use the purse organizer you bought. If you have shelf space, you can store them on the shelf. Organize according to size and color. Group the larger daytime bags together, then medium-size bags, and then put the clutches together. Make sure you can see everything and that nothing is getting crushed. The goal here is to keep only the bags that you actually use and to have everything organized so that you can easily switch purses when you change outfits or want to trade your day bag for an evening clutch.

**Collate jewelry.** Gather your jewelry—from all the pouches, plastic bags, travel cases, your nightstand, and your bathroom—and find one place to keep all of it, whether it is in the hanging jewelry organizer you just bought or a sizable jewelry box that can house all of your trinkets. You want to have your jewelry in one organized, easily accessible spot. No more wasting time untangling necklace chains or looking for the mate to an earring. Take the time now to untangle, pair off, and smartly store your jewelry in a way that is most functional for you.

**Fine-tune.** Then find a place for anything else left in your wardrobe—undergarments, socks, scarves and wraps, swimsuits, even hats. Most of these items will work best in a bureau drawer or neatly on a shelf. Again, organize and pair off these items neatly according to category and color.

Now, how do you feel? Take a look in your newly organized, cleaned-out, and clutter-free closet. You'll never have to root through messy piles again or get stressed in the morning because you have "nothing" to wear. Investing the time this weekend will save you time down the road. Plus, everything in your closet is now guaranteed to make you look and feel like your absolute best, most confident, sexiest self!

**Keep it neat.** The only catch is that now you need to maintain your beautiful new closet. Remember how great it feels to be organized and on top of your game, and make a promise to yourself that you will never let your closet get out of control again. Don't worry—it's much easier to maintain than it is to do another overhaul.

## TIPS FOR MAINTAINING YOUR CLOSET

- Hang, fold, or store every item and shoe every time you undress.
- Don't impulse shop. Put an item on hold, go home, and evaluate your needs before you purchase it.
- If you buy anything new, toss the item it is replacing.
- Take stock of every item before you get dressed. If anything has changed (fit, condition, etc.) and it is no longer a perfect 10, toss it.
- Consider any big changes—new job, new home, new city—and whether your wardrobe is still appropriate.
- Do a once-over at the change of every season to take stock, evaluate, and toss anything that doesn't make the cut.

It takes only 30 seconds to hang up your clothing and put your shoes back in the right place. Why just toss them back into the closet or, worse, into a laundry heap on the floor? Today, make a pact with yourself to hang, refold, and restore any worn or washed item as soon as you are done with it. We know you can afford ✓ the 30 seconds for your sanity. Can't you? Do this for the next 21 days in a row, it will become second nature, and you will have formed a positive new habit that will last a lifetime!

The other promise you must make (and believe us, now that the not-great items from your wardrobe are gone, you won't want it any other way) is that the only pieces you will *add* to your wardrobe going forward are perfect 10s. Every ✓ time you shop, consider the eight criteria for the closet cleanout for any item you are thinking about buying. If a garment or an accessory or footwear doesn't meet all the criteria, it is not a 10, and it does not belong in your closet. Doing this will allow you to manage your closet so well that it will never get out of control again!

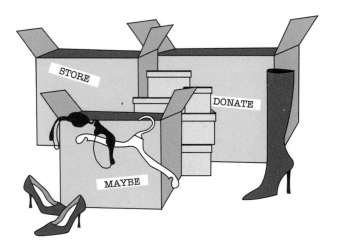

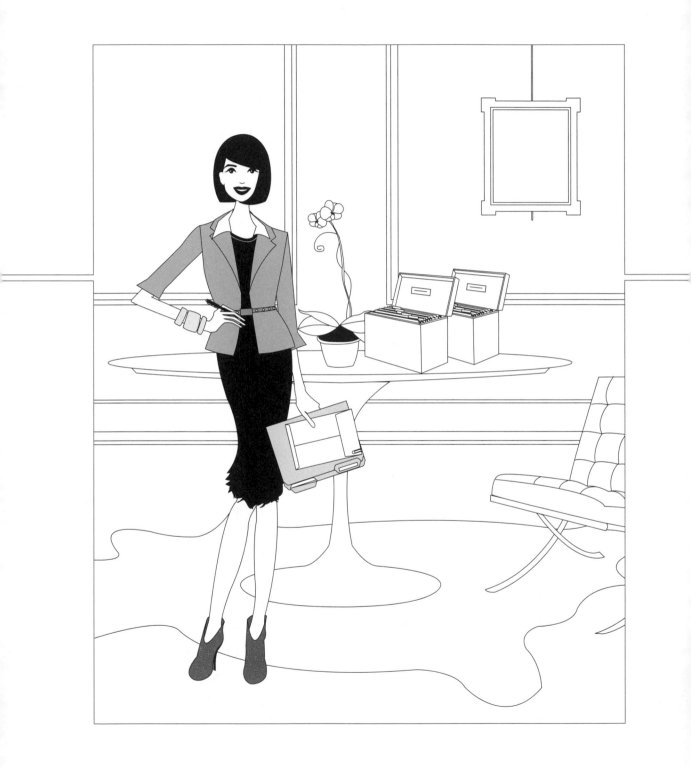

# *Chapter Eight*
# Clutter Makeover

When was the last time you cleaned out your files? Are you thinking, "*What* files?" You're not alone. According to the Small Business Administration, 80 percent of filed papers are never looked at again. How about the last time you went through that stack of unread or old magazines? Or really took a look at what you are storing (ahem, hoarding) in your home? One Boston marketing firm found that the average American wastes 55 minutes a day looking for things he knows are there but can't find. And according to researchers at UCLA's Center on Everyday Lives of Families, just 25 percent of garages can be used for cars—the other 75 percent are filled with *stuff.*

It's very easy, we know, to accumulate and accumulate without even realizing you are doing it. You don't have to be a shopaholic to end up with more than you ✓ need. Somehow, the stuff just ends up there—in the drawer, in the closet, under the bed. Unless we stay on top of it, the amount of unnecessary junk that ends up cluttering up our homes and our lives can get seriously out of control.

If you've already achieved the closet makeover in Chapter 7, you're now enjoying the freedom and functionality of a decluttered and organized closet—and you can see how easily this same technique could be applied anywhere in your home.

This weekend is your opportunity to do just that. You are going to clean out and pare down all the "stuff" you have been storing (or hoarding), for whatever reason. The longer you live someplace, the more you fill it up. If there is space, junk will come. Even if there isn't space, somehow we make room! Crazy, we know.

Just like when you cleaned out your closet, you will notice that there are items in your home that are perfectly fine—you just don't need them. These are harder to part with because, really, what's the reason to toss them? Your sanity, that's the reason! Ninety percent of Americans admit that disorganization at home or work has a negative impact on their lives—and 65 percent of those people said it specifically affects their state of mind.

Over the course of the weekend, you will purge all of your extraneous junk—everything from unnecessary paperwork to outdated sports equipment. Yes, you will go through everything. Get ready to declutter!

## ☾ FRIDAY NIGHT

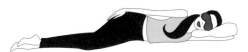

Don't feel overwhelmed: Some of your "stuff" is more obvious and easier to part with. To get started, we want you to tackle the clutter that is a no-brainer—outdated magazines, newspapers, and catalogs. If there is a newer edition than the one you are holding, the issue in your hand is outdated. Last month's *Vogue,* or even yesterday's newspaper, is outdated. As for catalogs, merchandise changes so often that companies won't necessarily have items in stock from previous catalogs. Tossing these booklets is easy—aim them right into the recycling bin.

This purge should be relaxing, not stressful. We are giving you permission to relieve yourself of the pressure of going through your ever-growing stack of

*Jill*

*I remember the first time I did a "round" and cleaned out the clothing in my closet. My close friends and discriminating accomplices, Shari and Brandee, sat on the bed with a bottle of champagne and gave me thumbs up or down for each outfit. I went nuts overnight, and all I wanted to do was clean out my whole apartment. I wanted everything organized and perfect. After I purged my closet, I moved on to my bathroom. I didn't realize how many items I had kept in my cabinets that I didn't use (let alone things that were expired). I feel like we are all obsessed with filling up space. I learned it is okay to have an empty shelf or an empty drawer. Space is good—you never know what could come into your life that might fit perfectly!*

*Dana*

*It might sound like I'm picking on my sister a little (I've mentioned her fridge and now her home), because she does tend to save everything (yes, she has clothing from high school stashed at my parents' house because she has no room in her apartment). Every time I visit, I see these massive piles of catalogs and magazines stacked on her desk, nightstand, and floor. She swears up and down that she is going to get to them, but each time I visit, the stacks have only grown bigger. I don't know what buried treasure she thinks she'll find in there! Maybe she will prove me wrong. I, on the other hand, don't so much as let a catalog enter my home. I take them straight from my mailbox to the recycling bin down my hall. I used to feel I needed to read every magazine under the sun just to keep up with everything new and cool. Now I am down to my three faves:* Elle, Vanity Fair, *and* Vogue. *I make sure I keep up with reading them as they come in.*

catalogs, newspapers, and magazines—just toss them all! Trust us. Don't even open them. If the stack is that high, we guarantee that nothing in there is worth your time. We'll let you in on a little secret: You're not missing anything! Really. You don't *need* anything in the catalogs (you'll get another one in your mailbox next week anyway), and you will likely see or hear about anything in the older magazines or newspapers somewhere else, too—whether on TV, in a store, through social media, or by gossiping with your best friend.

If there are articles or stories you'd like to read eventually, clip them from the magazines or pull them from the paper stack and save them in a folder that you can put away in a drawer or keep on your bedside table. But you don't need that huge stack sitting there. You will probably never sit down one day and read *all* those magazines and newspapers or thumb through *all* those catalogs. Everything moves so fast these days that if you don't see it/read it/buy it immediately, it becomes outdated and therefore unnecessary.

Now literally take your piles and get them out of your home tonight. Let them go. You are missing nothing. Bring them to the recycling bin in your apartment building or house and out of your range of vision. You should notice a vast improvement already. Good job for tonight. Enjoy your already increased space. Are you smiling yet? Take a breath and feel good that you've made a significant start to your weekend. Settle into your evening and relax over a nice dinner—or if you ate before you began, maybe it's time for dessert!

Get a good night's rest, and we'll have more fun tomorrow!

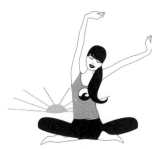

## SATURDAY MORNING

This morning we focus on another project involving paper, but one that takes a bit more concentration than simply recycling most of it. It's time to go through your paperwork—bills, documents, receipts—and set up a filing system that works for you. Believe us, when you are finished, you will feel 10 times better!

This is going to require a little patience and a lot of sitting, so before you get started, enjoy a nice breakfast and get motivated to purge. If you have file folders and a file box (or file drawer or cabinet) that are in good condition and usable, collect them now and have them handy. If not, make a quick trip to Staples or Office Depot and purchase these organizational supplies and maybe even a shredder—you're gonna need it!

What's in your pile of papers? We're picturing receipts from the dawn of time, cable bills from when you first moved in, and tax returns from the '80s. Are we close?

We realize it can be very confusing to know what to keep and file for tax purposes, for example, and what's safe to throw away. Let's clear that up. Follow these guidelines for what needs to be saved and for how long:

**Tax returns.** Keep these for 6 years. This includes completed tax forms 1040, 1099s, and W-2 forms. After 6 years, you can throw away the oldest one (that is now 7 years old) and keep the most recent ones.

**Receipts.** If you deduct anything you purchased, these receipts need to be kept for 3 years. Any backup info, receipts, or paperwork you have that was included on your tax return must be filed for 3 years. Each year, as you file a new return, you can purge the oldest batch of receipts (that is now 4 years old). If you are not deducting the purchase, the receipt is garbage as soon as the transaction shows up on your credit card statement and you are committed to keeping the purchase. (Hold on to the receipt if you think you might return the item, and read it to see if, and for how long, the store accepts returns. After that returns period, you can toss the receipt.) For any big-ticket items, it is always a good idea to keep the receipt and warranty in case you need repairs or want to resell.

**Bills.** These do not need to be kept at all, unless you are deducting anything on them for tax purposes. If you are deducting any expenses from these bills, they must be kept for 3 years. If you are not deducting, once you get a bill and pay it, you no longer need to save it. For example, cable bills, phone bills, utility bills, and credit card statements not being deducted can all be tossed once paid.

**Deeds.** These should be kept and filed. If you own a house and/or a car, this paperwork must be stored somewhere safe for the duration that you are the owner. This paperwork will be necessary when and if you sell the item.

**Home improvement records.** Keep all paperwork, receipts, and canceled checks pertaining to home-improvement work you have done. When you want to sell your home, these will be proof of how much the improvement is worth.

**Canceled checks.** If a check pertains to something being deducted for tax purposes, save the canceled check for 3 years. If you are not using the checks to deduct anything on your taxes, save the canceled checks for 1 year.

**Bank statements.** These should be kept for 3 years, and then you can toss them.

**ATM receipts.** These can be tossed as soon as the record of the transaction appears on your bank statement.

**Paycheck stubs.** Hold on to these just until you receive your W-2 form. If all is in order, you can toss them.

**Airline tickets and boarding passes.** Unless the flight is a tax deductible expense, you can toss tickets and passes right after your trip or as soon as the miles appear in your frequent-flier account. If you are deducting the expense, save just the ticket receipt for 3 years.

**IRA contribution slips.** Save these and Form 8606 (what you file when you make a nondeductible IRA contribution). You'll need these when you retire to make sure you are not taxed again for any after-tax contributions.

**Investment information.** Keep paperwork that documents any investment transaction for the duration that you own the investment—stock, mutual fund, etc.—and for 6 years after you sell it. Keep this with your tax return info.

We know this is a lot of paper to go through, especially if you haven't purged in years, don't do your filing regularly, or don't have everything in one place. But it must be done. You have promised yourself this weekend to make over this area of your life—and it is a big one. Trust us, once you have this situation under control, when it comes to tax time (or anytime you need to locate important financial info), you will be a happy camper. As you know from the other makeovers

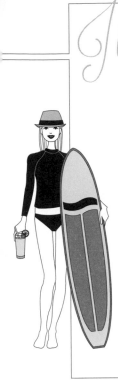

*Jill* *I am still a pen-and-paper kind of girl. I love folders—and labeling them! I also love writing lists on paper and being able to physically cross things off when I'm done. This is my way of staying organized. However, I only keep papers that are must-haves, and I try to be digitally organized whenever possible. I am not technologically savvy, but it's easier and easier these days to save digital files, and it keeps me clutter free.*

*Dana* *I hate clutter, so I constantly file and clean out my files as I go. Everything is neatly organized and all together in one file box. (This "box" started out as an accordion folder and has somehow grown to an actual box with hanging file folders—all neatly labeled, of course.) I know exactly where to look if I need to reference anything in my paperwork. I have some folders that are labeled and that I no longer use because I get most of my bills and statements electronically now.*

in this book, once you get a system in place, you will never have to start from scratch again!

**Protect yourself.** As you go through each piece of paper (yes, every one!), determine whether it can go or it needs to be kept and filed properly. If the paper is disposable and doesn't have private information on it (credit card number, Social Security number, bank account number, etc.), start stuffing a garbage bag. If it does have important private information, put it in a pile for the shredding party you will have later. If you feel more comfortable shredding *everything* you discard, by all means, do. About 8.6 million households had at least one person over the age of 12 experience identity theft in 2010, according to the Bureau of Justice Statistics. US households lost $13.3 billion because of it in that same year. To avoid becoming a victim of identity theft, the Federal Trade Commission recommends shredding charge receipts, copies of credit applications, insurance forms, physician statements, checks and bank statements, expired charge cards that you're discarding, and credit offers you get in the mail.

**Get organized!** For the documents and papers you will keep, now's the time to institute your working filing system. Be sure to label your folders and start filing as you go. File everything in its appropriate folder in date order starting in January and going in calendar order through December. This way, when you go through all your paperwork to file your taxes, you will know where everything is and it will be easy to locate.

Once your "keeper" paperwork is filed, it's time to shred! This will feel great. Now that you have done the hard work, take a time-out for a little brainless catharsis. You obviously don't want anyone to get hold of paperwork that has your personal information, so put everything that falls in that category through the shredder. Throw the shreds in the garbage with the rest of the trash and take out the big bag of what was all of your unnecessary paperwork. Get it out of the house and see how light you feel.

Now is the time to promise yourself that you will file your paperwork every single month. If you still get paper bills, statements, etc., in the mail, immediately file everything in its appropriate file folder, which should be individually labeled to reflect the contents—credit card, bank, paycheck, and so on. If you have graduated to online banking and bill paying, keep all of your records filed appropriately as well. You can create folders in your e-mail account to label and store each e-mail record in its appropriate folder—credit card bills, bank statements, frequent-flier miles, and so on. The perfect time to do this is when you pay your monthly bills. So if it's the 1st of the month or the 15th, set aside half an hour after you pay your bills to file everything in the appropriate folder (a well-maintained system will probably require less than 30 minutes). The stress of dealing with unexpected bills and random receipts will disappear.

You did it! You should be so proud. Take a break, nourish yourself with a healthy lunch, and walk around the block to get the blood flowing in your legs again. We know it was a lot to ask to sit and go through a lifetime of paperwork. But now you won't have to do it again!

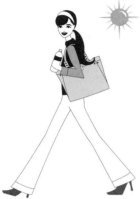# SATURDAY AFTERNOON

Your next project is going to be more fun and a lot less tedious than the paperwork situation this morning. Are you ready to go? This afternoon you pare down and get rid of anything else you have been storing (ahem, hoarding) in your house that you don't need but never really saw a reason to get rid of.

Pare down your "collections." Most times, we don't realize that we are creating a collection of junk because it happens so gradually. For example: dishes. Perhaps you got a set of dishes when you went away to college or first moved out on your own. Quite likely, some of those broke, or you never had a full set, or you grew out of the style/color/pattern, so at some point you bought a different set but never threw away the old ones. Why would you? They still work, right? And then maybe you got married, or moved again, and got another full set of dishes—quite possibly everyday dishes *and* fancy china or an elegant set for entertaining, and yet you still held on to your original dishes from college or your first place.

Why? They're certainly still good, but in reality they are taking up valuable storage/shelf space in your home. Truthfully, if you don't use them, they are just, well, clutter!

Decide which dishes you do use, put those aside, and start to pile up the ones you don't. You can donate the extra dishes to charity or give them away to someone just starting out on his or her own. If you have full sets that are in great shape, but you don't love the style anymore, you can try to resell them on eBay or Craigslist.

Another example of something that can easily accumulate: vases. We're not talking about the ones you purposefully bought or that were given to you as a gift and have special meaning. We are talking generic glass vases that come in all shapes and sizes from the florist when you get a flower delivery, or from center-pieces that you took home after weddings or events, or the empty food jars and bottles you saved to use for flowers. Yes, those.

It's funny how this happens. You get flowers, and then after they die, you wash the vase and put it away with the others, without even looking or realizing how many of the exact same ones you already have! Unless one cracks or breaks, there is really no reason to throw them out. Right? But, ah, there is a reason (actually, three): You don't need the clutter, you will never use *all* of them, and they are taking up valuable storage space that you might put to better use.

So here's the plan. Take them all out of the cabinet or closet and set them on a table. Go through them one by one. Get rid of duplicates (unless you like a particular size or style and may use two at a time). Get rid of the shapes you don't like and won't use again. Decide how many, realistically, you need to keep, which ones you will actually use, and how many you have room to store.

We know that vases and containers come in all shapes and sizes, so you might need a variety (we love the idea of filling a home with flowers!). Keep enough so

*Jill* *Speaking of vases, a few weeks ago I got a call from my mother: "I just got rid of 10 vases." I asked, "How many did you have?" The answer? Twenty-five! Why would anyone need 25 vases? The answer: You don't. I try to keep this in mind every time I get flowers. I have stopped accumulating vases. I have just the right amount that I need, and any new ones go right to the recycling bin as soon as the flowers wilt.*

*Dana* *Somehow over the years, I seem to have amassed a collection of glass vases. I have a variety of sizes and shapes and am pretty good about not keeping too many duplicates, but I can always use a clean-out. I sometimes have visions of having a dinner party at a long table with flowers at every person's table setting—but then I remember I need a house and long dining table first! See how easy it is to make excuses to keep stuff around?*

that you can have a few arrangements around the house at the same time. Even better—before you put vases back in the cabinet, leave one or two out and reward yourself for clearing the clutter with fresh blooms this afternoon! Make your home pretty and your vases useful!

Remember the recycling bin where you took all your magazines, newspapers, and catalogs last night? Well, the one next to it is for glass! Take all the vases you are not keeping down the hall or into the garage and place them in the appropriate bin.

Bed, bath, and . . . beyond. Now head into your bedroom and bathroom for the next area awaiting help: old or extra bedding, sheets, blankets, and towels. How many of these do you really need? We know how it happens: A sheet or pillow-case gets ripped or stained, so you toss it out and buy a whole new sheet set, but you still keep the rest of the old set. It's like having one sock when you've lost the other in the dryer. (Speaking of which, toss those single socks, too!) You will never use that partial sheet set again. We promise! It's sometimes hard to rationalize throwing out sheets when there's nothing wrong with them, but honestly, will you use just a top or bottom sheet or just one pillowcase? Probably not. It will simply sit there taking up space in the vortex of your linen closet, never to be used again, while at the same time, you can't rationalize tossing it because, well, there's nothing wrong with it.

We are giving you permission now to toss the partial sheet sets. Now, if you are able to legitimately use them, great! (And we mean really use them, such as cutting them up for cleaning rags, using them as padding to store artwork or fragile items, or sewing them into a Halloween costume for your child.) But if they are never going to be transformed into anything other than clutter, dump 'em. Go for it! Doesn't a clutter-free home sound so much better than hoarding things you just feel bad about tossing—or didn't even consider tossing? Just like the situation with the vases, it's easy to go on autopilot and follow the instinct to put them away. You may not have paused to think whether to keep or toss. Your default action (don't feel bad, most everyone is set up this way) is to keep everything.

We often don't think of cleaning out as we live through our day to day. We just keep, store, and hoard, until it gets to the point where we must purge. This

*Jill* *Again, I am throwing my mother under the bus, but when you open the linen closet in my childhood home (where my parents still live), everything falls out. She still has the pink flowered sheets from when I was 9 and sleeping in a twin bed (meanwhile, they don't have a twin bed anymore). There are new beautiful sheet sets in the linen closet (at least three, which is probably more than they need), and I don't think she uses them because there is so much clutter in the way. She loves the pink flowered ones because they were my favorite when I was younger (so sweet), but I have new favorites now, so let's use those!*

*Dana* *As soon as one of my towels starts looking dingy, I replace it with a new one. (Meaning the old one literally goes in the garbage.) I love the look and feel of new towels. However, I just recently got rid of some spare partial sheet sets. I had been hanging on to two flat sheets—from separate sets—and a couple of random pillowcases that had threads and strings hanging from them but were still usable. I don't know what I was thinking (perhaps a guest would use them someday?), but one day I did a massive cleanout, came to my senses, and tossed all of them!*

purging is a valuable lesson, and once you learn it, you will be able to revamp your thinking so that you consider everything that comes into your home before mindlessly stashing it away in a closet or cabinet or, heaven forbid, under the bed!

Just because someone buys you a gift is no reason to keep it. And if you purchase something new—theoretically to replace something you already have— toss the old one. Do you really need both? We thought not.

Blankets are another item that tends to accumulate. We're sure you don't need all of those. Keep the number you need for all the beds in your home and maybe one or two spares for houseguests, if you entertain. Donate the rest. Yes, it's hard to part with these when there's nothing wrong with them. This is your clutter makeover, however, and what's wrong is that you have too much clutter! A donation of blankets to a homeless shelter is always appreciated, and there is no way you are going to feel bad eliminating them when you know they'll go to good use—way better use than sitting in your closet. Right? Thank you.

Towels, too. Toss the ones that are not in great condition and start fresh with new ones. This will not only make you happy—as we know, fresh towels and new bedding always make us feel great, but it will also reduce your clutter and keep your home items up to par with your wardrobe—a perfect 10. Why would you accept anything less? You deserve the best!

Again, keep only the perfect-10 towels (don't put the old ones back on the shelf because you think you might "need" them someday—you won't). Keep only the quantity you need for every member of your household, depending on how often you do laundry, and a couple of spares for guests. We'll leave that number up to you, but be realistic and honest about what you actually need and use.

Okay, we've given you a couple of examples here about how, what, why, and where clutter comes from. Now it's your turn to do a once-over of your entire house. Don't worry! It sounds more daunting than it is.

## CLUTTER CLEANOUT

Useless/meaningless tchotchkes ✓

~~Old/broken appliances~~

Costume jewelry you don't wear

Inherited items that aren't your style

Gifts that aren't your taste

CDs that have been imported into your iTunes

Books that you have read and don't intend to read again

Schoolwork/books/papers from childhood/college

Random memorabilia

Cards/notes with no sentimental value

We don't want you to get rid of all of your earthly possessions. We do want you to go through every closet, cabinet, and possible storage space and take stock of what you might be unwittingly collecting. Accumulating extra junk happens almost by accident. Especially when you haven't moved in years, it seems like there's no real reason to go through and clean out. Well, the reason is this: It's your dedicated weekend to make over your home and eliminate the clutter. Good enough reason? Great!

You have all day tomorrow to finish this project, so don't overdo it today. When you feel satisfied with what you've accomplished so far, declare yourself finished, take out the remaining trash, make a drive to the donation center to unload the blankets (and anything else donation-worthy), and buy yourself some pretty flowers (using those vases that you "had" to keep!) to celebrate your almost clutter-free home.

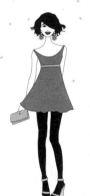

## SATURDAY NIGHT

Do something nice for yourself this evening, whether it is going out for dinner, to a movie, to a party, or just relaxing at home. We're sure you will sleep well knowing you are firmly on the road to accomplishing your weekend mission.

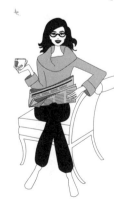

## SUNDAY

This morning, nourish yourself with a healthy breakfast and revel in your almost clutter-free home. You should have your list (even if it's just a mental list) of what's left to clean out and unload today. We have more suggestions in case these are conspicuously missing from your to-do list: sporting equipment and old electronic gadgets.

Let's start with sporting equipment. We always think there

*Jill* *I moved into a building in the city that has a rooftop pool. It is a lap pool, and when I moved in, I said, "I am going to swim every day." So, of course, I went to a sporting goods store and bought the best goggles, swim cap, and flippers and set myself up for swimming success. I swam once. For a half hour. And now I have enough equipment to start a summer camp. I could have bought a pair of Jimmy Choos for what I spent on gear!*

*Dana* *I used to play tennis, inline skate, ski, and ice-skate, enough that I invested in my own equipment. I kept all of this "stuff" around way past the point that these activities were no longer part of my weekly, monthly, or even yearly repertoire. By the time I sold my tennis racquet and ski equipment (both from high school, mind you) at a yard sale, I was in my thirties. Okay, embarrassing, but at least I got rid of them. The racquet didn't take up much room, but the skis and poles were pretty big. I loved those skis—they were green Rossignols with matching poles—but skis are not even made in that shape anymore! Now if I am going to play tennis, I can always borrow a racquet, and if I go skiing, I will rent equipment (from this century, LOL). Admittedly, I do still have my Rollerblades and ice skates. I don't use the Rollerblades often, but the occasion has come up, and they still work. As for the ice skates, my niece and nephew had an ice-skating birthday party last year, so, of course, I skated, and I look forward to skating with them as often as I can. I think I'll hold on to those. And, no, they are not outdated!*

might be that one time that someone will invite us to play tennis, or go inline skating, or skiing, or [*fill in the sport here*]. If you don't participate in these activities of your own accord, don't worry about that one-time what-if scenario. Could it happen? Yes. Will it? Maybe. Can you worry about it at that time and either borrow, rent, or buy new equipment if it is something you plan on doing often? Absolutely.

Here's the thing: Sporting equipment gets outdated. If you haven't played in years but are still holding on to your old racquet, chances are good that you will not want to use it should the opportunity arise. Equipment also tends to take up a lot of valuable storage real estate. Sure, you could fit a tennis racquet in the closet, but add to that the skates, skis, boots, etc., and you have gotten yourself a collection, accidental or otherwise. So whatever you don't regularly use—meaning you can't remember the last time you played and it was not relatively recently—toss! Or rather, in this case, it might be nice to donate.

Now for the electronics. We all know how fast these items get outdated. It's hard to keep up. The general rule, though, is that as soon as you replace something—whether it is a computer, a cell phone, a camera, or an iPod—the old one is pretty much moot.

Again, that little voice in your head may be saying that it's still working, what if you need it someday, or it was so expensive. Well, yes, but you have the newer, faster, cleaner, better model, correct? Just like your clothing, bedding, and sports equipment, once an electronic gadget goes out of your rotation, it is over. Yes, *over*. You can store it, but we promise you are never using it again. If your new cell phone breaks, will you buy a newer one or dust off the old, outdated model? Thought so. Okay, enough said.

What to do with old electronics? Don't toss them in the trash. According to an article from Rodale.com, e-waste is not like traditional garbage: "Electronics contain heavy metals and toxic chemicals, such as lead, mercury, cadmium, and brominated flame retardants (these have been linked to thyroid problems and learning disabilities)." We don't want these chemicals leaching from landfills into groundwater or incinerated into toxic air pollutants. Instead, recycle old electronics. Or better yet, if any items are in working order, donating is the way to go.

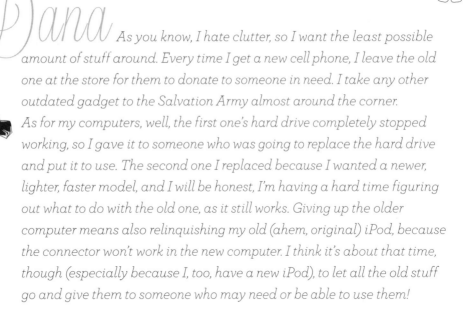

*Jill* *I held on to my first Mac computer for as long as I could. I needed to upgrade for work, but it was hard to part with my original white Mac. My brother, Jonathan, started a charity called KidCare that works with underprivileged children. He was able to give my old computer to Scott, the student he was mentoring. Scott said to him, "This is the best gift I have ever gotten." This made me smile, and I am so happy that computer found a new home.*

*Dana* *As you know, I hate clutter, so I want the least possible amount of stuff around. Every time I get a new cell phone, I leave the old one at the store for them to donate to someone in need. I take any other outdated gadget to the Salvation Army almost around the corner. As for my computers, well, the first one's hard drive completely stopped working, so I gave it to someone who was going to replace the hard drive and put it to use. The second one I replaced because I wanted a newer, lighter, faster model, and I will be honest, I'm having a hard time figuring out what to do with the old one, as it still works. Giving up the older computer means also relinquishing my old (ahem, original) iPod, because the connector won't work in the new computer. I think it's about that time, though (especially because I, too, have a new iPod), to let all the old stuff go and give them to someone who may need or be able to use them!*

Most schools would be thrilled to receive an older-model working computer. All of the cell phone companies would be happy to take your old mobile phone and donate it to people to use for emergency calls to 911. Your old, usable camera, iPod, speakers, clock radio, DVD player, TV, etc., can go to a local donation center for a tax write-off. Just make sure you wipe any device of all of your personal info, contacts, photos, music, and files before you donate. If you are worried about purging all of your personal electronic data, use a DoD certified wiping service like this one: www.data-destruction.com/dod_certified_destruction.html.

Two sources to find places to donate or recycle electronics are www.epa.gov/osw/conserve/materials/ecycling/donate.htm and e-stewards.org/find-a-recycler. Or sell old electronics here: www.usell.com/why-usell.htm.

By the end of today, you should have gone through your entire house and decluttered it of the junk you no longer need, no longer use, and no longer have room for. Now it's time to make a pact with yourself that you will carefully consider everything that comes into your home. Just because an object comes in the front door does not mean it needs to find a storage space in a nook or cranny or, worse, pile up in plain view. You have the power to decide what stays and what goes—every day. Use that power.

It's just like the rule you made for yourself about buying new clothes—if the object is not a perfect 10, it doesn't deserve or get a space in your closet.

Now, if you have a husband and/or children, you will have more than just your own stuff to contend with. Your husband might be holding on to things that are clearly clutter to you, and likewise your kids will have a collection of toys, stuffed animals, and arts and crafts projects.

Start by offering to help your husband purge his items, the same way that you did. Walk him through the process and get rid of much as is reasonable. Do the same with your kids' things. As they grow and accumulate new toys, they will likely not use the old ones. Do a cleanout with them, helping them evaluate what they use and what items they

## **6** WAYS TO KEEP YOUR CAR CLUTTER FREE

1. Empty the trash every day—food wrappers/water bottles/coffee cups.

2. Take out extra clothing you brought for the day—jacket/sweater/pair of flats.

3. Take the mail/paperwork with you and sort it at home to stay on top of it.

4. Keep kids' toys/games to a minimum and store in a bin.

5. Keep music CDs organized and in a case.

6. Whatever you brought with you in the morning, take out in the evening.

want to keep. Giving their old toys, dolls, and games to children in need is a great way to teach youngsters about giving back.

After you and your household get rid of everything that is not essential and useful, figure out a system to organize the stuff that remains so that these items are not creating an environment of clutter. Store your papers in filing cabinets, magazines in a rack, and the kids' toys in toy bins. Keep your desk, counters, and tables clear of everything except what you use for decorative purposes.

So, to review, keep only the reading materials that are current and that you plan on reading (truly make a point and take the time to actually read them), and commit to toss the ones that aren't current and that you won't read. File only the paperwork that needs to be saved for tax or resale purposes, and toss the documents that don't need retaining (see pages 131–32). Keep only the dishes, vases, bedding, sports equipment, electronic gadgets, and [*fill in the blank here*] that you will and do use. Donate the rest accordingly.

That should be pretty clear and easy. Now that you have done the work and you know the drill, keep it up. It feels great to have a clutter-free home, doesn't it? Thought so. You can do this. We have faith in you. Congrats on this huge weekend project. Enjoy your Sunday evening. You deserve it!

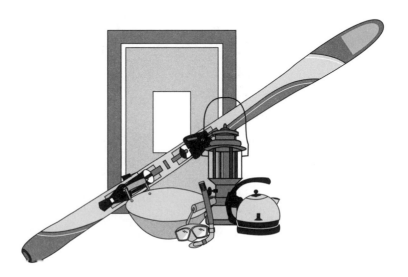

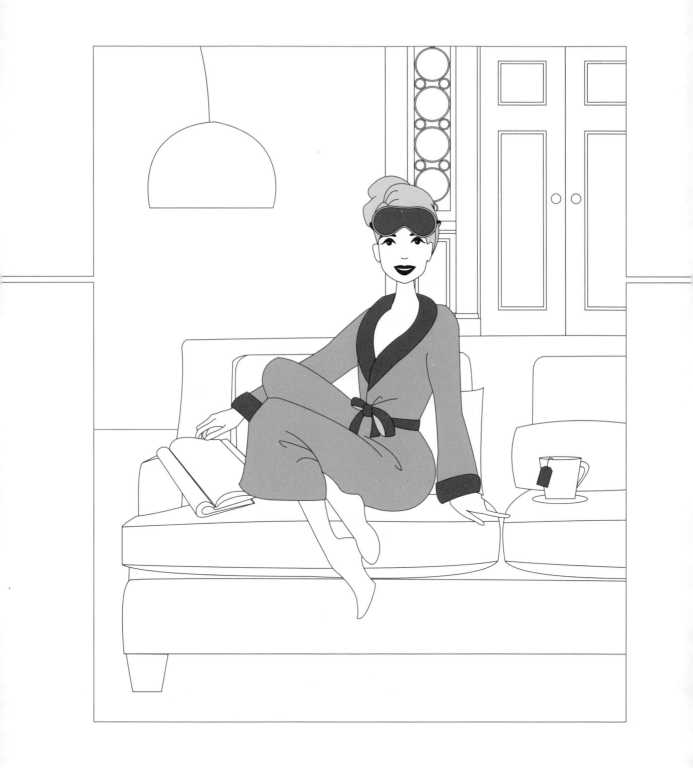

# Chapter Nine

# Relaxation Makeover

Y ou've already done a lot of work on your body, your mind, and your home—so this makeover should be a well-deserved piece of cake. Well, in theory, that is. This weekend is all about relaxing and creating a spalike ambience in your home. Although this may sound divine, shutting off the outside world can be very difficult for most people. Are you prepared to detach yourself from your phone, computer, and TV for a bit? Do you think you can relax and retreat from the world?

Whether we are e-mailing, texting, or tweeting, we are all so reliant on our electronic devices to keep us up-to-date and in contact all the time that we forget what it's like to have peace and quiet. Sixty percent of people don't go an hour without checking their phone, according to the Mobile Mindset Study. It's no surprise that younger adults are more addicted, with 63 percent of women and 73 percent of men ages 18 to 34 checking their phones at least every hour.

People are staying connected 24/7, whether in bed, in the car, or even on the toilet (yes, 40 percent admitted to checking their phones while visiting the restroom!). A study conducted by the International Center for Media and the Public Agenda asked 200 students at the University of Maryland, College Park, to abstain from using all media for 24 hours. Not only were most students unwilling to participate, but those who did were unable to function without their media links to the world.

But turning off and tuning out are worthy and necessary. The University of Maryland Medical Center found that relaxation techniques can reduce symptoms or improve outcomes of many conditions, such as high blood pressure, diabetes, insomnia, and irritable bowel syndrome. You deserve this mini-break, this weekend to chill, recharge, and reboot. It's totally okay to drop out for these couple of days and take care of *you*. It's often hard to remember amid our busy lives, with all of the people counting on us—partners, kids, bosses, co-workers, friends, family—that we have to take care of ourselves first and foremost. Oftentimes, we actually end up last on that list, if we're on it at all.

That's about to change. This weekend you will spend time relaxing and pampering. And you are going to promise yourself to find the time to incorporate some of the "spa" feeling in your busy day-to-day life.

Get your responsibilities (kids and husband or partner, if you have them) sorted for the weekend so you can take "me" time, guilt free. If you can arrange for your kids to stay over at Grandma and Grandpa's house or another relative's, or at one of their friend's homes, great! If not, maybe you can give your husband an IOU for keeping your kids (and him) out of the house for a good portion of the weekend. Plan some activities or organize playdates for the children so they are happily occupied and not occupying you! If family members do end up at home with you for part of the weekend, explain nicely that Mommy is off duty this weekend and that all inquiries and needs should be directed to Dad. It is fair to let them know that if Mommy's bathroom or bedroom door is shut, she does not want to be disturbed. You are entitled to your privacy as much as anybody. Ready? Let's get started!

# ☾ FRIDAY NIGHT

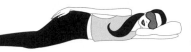

It's Friday night. The workweek is over. You have nowhere to be until Monday morning. Sound good? You have cleared this weekend of plans and responsibilities (to the best of your ability), so no one will be expecting anything from you or of you. Aah, freedom.

**Shut down—responsibly.** Your first task is to shut off your cell phone, your computer, and your TV. Ideally, these will be left off for the entire weekend to really evoke the spa ambience in your home—nothing ringing, no extraneous noise, no pinging e-mails to respond to. If you are tempted just by the sight of these objects, do your best to keep them out of view—put your cell phone in a drawer, along with the TV remote; drape a pretty scarf over your computer and another over the TV to disguise them and make your surroundings a little softer and cozier.

Should you need to use your electronic devices, please apply discretion as to how much. If you are concerned with shutting off completely for the weekend and bothered by the thought "What if someone really needs me?" then place an out-of-office/vacation responder on your e-mail and change your voice mail to indicate that you are unavailable until Monday morning and to contact [*fill in the blank here*] in case of an emergency. You are taking a time-out to decompress, but that doesn't mean you have to completely isolate yourself. Knowing

## OUR FAVORITE TOP 10 RELAXING ALBUMS

1. Carly Simon: *Greatest Hits Live*
2. Carole King: *Tapestry*
3. Cat Stevens: *Greatest Hits*
4. Eagles: *The Very Best of Eagles*
5. James Taylor: *Greatest Hits*
6. Ray LaMontagne: *Gossip in the Grain*
7. Sade: *The Best of Sade*
8. Steely Dan: *A Decade of Steely Dan*
9. Toni Braxton: *The Essential Toni Braxton*
10. Van Morrison: *Astral Weeks*

that you won't be disturbed—but that you can still be reached in case of emergency—will help you relax and settle into a peaceful state of mind.

Begin to see your home as a relaxing place, not a hectic one. This weekend you are going to design your environment. Don't worry if you don't have all the supplies right now. We'll fix that tomorrow.

**Set the mood.** This evening, if you have dimmers on the lighting, dim the lights lower than you normally keep them. Or try using table or floor lamps instead of overhead lighting. If you have candles, light a few with soothing scents. Put on mellow music—the opposite of what is on your workout playlist! If you don't have relaxing music on your iPod, you have permission to tune your TV to one of the all-music channels (easy listening, of course!) or to stream Pandora. Choose a genre that you like. It doesn't have to be classical to be relaxing. Whether you enjoy jazz, R&B, soul, or oldies, pick what soothes you.

The mood is set, and now it's up to you what you'd like to do for the rest of the night. Dine leisurely over a nutritious, healthy "spa" dinner—perhaps a piece of grilled fish with brown rice and steamed or sautéed veggies, or a delicious green salad with a piece of grilled chicken, or a light veggie stir-fry with tofu over rice. Luxuriate in a long, hot bath, curl up and start a new book, catch up on your favorite magazine, or all of the above! It's sort of a strange feeling when you start to let yourself unwind, let go, and realize you have nothing else to do. Isn't it? You might find you are relaxed enough to fall asleep early and catch up on some z's.

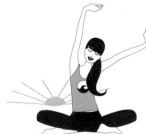

# SATURDAY MORNING

Good morning! We hope you slept well after a relaxing evening. Today will be more of the same. In fact, this whole weekend is going to be about learning how to unwind and take care of yourself.

If you don't have to turn on your phone, computer, or TV, don't! Escape for as long as you can into the blissful silence that has taken over your home. Feel free to lounge, read, eat, bathe, or anything else you enjoy. You have nowhere you need to be.

*Jill*  I sleep with my BlackBerry. I am not kidding. Well, it is on the side table next to my bed, but it is accessible at all times and always on. Sometimes I wish I wasn't such a slave to it. I am working on separating myself, but in the meantime, I have a few rules I live by: The phone is never on the table while I am eating dinner, I try not to type while walking on the streets of New York (I hate when people typing bump into me), and I give myself 1 hour a night when I put the phone on silent and watch a movie or watch TV without interruption. Following my rules is hard, but it is the only thing that keeps me sane (or at least partially sane!).

*Dana*  I'm on e-mail for work all the time, and, of course, mail comes to my iPhone. There's nothing I love more than making the decision to not respond to any work e-mails after 7:00 p.m. during the week or over the entire weekend. Mind you, I get e-mails at all hours of the day and night, so if I let myself, I'd never get the chance to shut off and take a break. After a while, I realized that nothing was going to happen if I didn't respond to an e-mail immediately, especially after normal business hours. And you know what? I was right!

**Stock up on soothers.** To make your home the ultimate spa experience, you might need a few supplies, if you don't have them already. When you're motivated to head outside (if you feel like moving at all!), consider putting the following on your shopping list:

*Candles.* Our advice is to buy all the same scent (if you are going to light more

# DIY *Masks and Scrubs*

## Oatmeal and Yogurt Face Mask

1 tablespoon oatmeal, finely ground

1 tablespoon live, organic, plain yogurt

A few drops of honey

In a small bowl, mix the oatmeal and yogurt together. Run a spoon under hot water for a minute. Then, with the hot spoon, add a few drops of honey and stir it into the oatmeal-yogurt mixture. Apply the mask to the face, leave on for 10 minutes, and then rinse off with warm water.

## Sugar Face Scrub

2 tablespoons sugar

3 tablespoons warm water

In a small bowl, stir the sugar into the warm water until the granules dissolve. Apply to the face and massage around on the skin. Rinse with warm water.

## Avocado, Coconut Milk, and Olive Oil Hair Mask

1 ripe avocado

½ cup coconut milk

3 teaspoons olive oil

In a small saucepan, mash the avocado. Add the coconut milk and olive oil and stir until mixed well. Heat the mask on the stove until warm. Apply the mask from the hair roots to the ends and massage into the scalp. Leave on for at least 30 minutes and then wash the hair.

## Salt or Sugar and Oil Body Scrub

1 cup salt or sugar
   (small granules for either)

½ cup oil (extra virgin coconut, almond, or olive oil)

5 drops of essential oil
   (optional, for scent purposes)

In a small bowl, mix the salt or sugar with the oil and add the essential oil, if desired. In the bath or shower, rub the mixture over your body in a circular motion either with your hands or a washcloth. Take extra time and care with dry areas such as the elbows and knees and the bottoms of the feet. Be gentle on the chest and neck area, where skin is thinner. Fully rinse when finished. The oil should leave you soft and moisturized.

than one at the same time in the same room) or a few complementary scents (all floral, for example). Lavender is known for its relaxing properties, so if you like the smell, this is always a good choice. Candles come in every fragrance from vanilla to jasmine and every fruit and herb in between. Some smell like the ocean, and some like fresh-cut grass. Choose a scent that is pleasing to *you,* but not too strong. Get enough candles to stage around your home. It's nice to have one, at least, in your living room and bathroom and on your nightstand. Having more than one in each room enhances the experience and might enable you to turn off the lights! For the healthiest and most environmentally friendly option, select candles with soy-based wax and lead-free wicks.

*Face mask.* If you bought a mask for your beauty makeover (Chapter 3), you are good to go. If you want to try a different mask, feel free to experiment. Make sure the one you purchase is appropriate for your skin type—dry, oily, sensitive, problem, aging or damaged, or normal. If you want to get adventurous, check out "DIY Masks and Scrubs" and make your very own homemade face mask out of all-natural food ingredients. Generally, DIY masks require just a few ingredients that you may already have in your fridge or that you can pick up this morning.

*Face scrub.* You should also have a scrub from the beauty makeover, but if you don't, you can easily purchase one now or play around with our homemade recipe on the opposite page. While you don't want to use anything rough (like body scrub) on your face, you can apply face scrub to your body. Simply make a double batch from scratch, or purchase additional product.

*Hair mask.* This is easily found in the store or made at home out of fresh ingredients (see the opposite page). Totally up to you. It may depend on how much you enjoy spending time in the kitchen!

*Body scrub.* This type of scrub is generally a little rougher than face scrub, as your skin is more delicate around the face and neck area. If you choose to make body scrub at home, try our version on the opposite page.

*Tea.* If you don't keep tea at home, buy yourself some now. Herbal or de-caffeinated tea is best, as the goal here is to relax and unwind. You can get loose tea if you want to brew it yourself, but tea bags are sufficient. As with candles, tea comes in a gazillion tea varieties, from fruity to floral to spicy. Pick up a box of your fave, or choose a few different flavors to try. Lots of companies package assorted flavors. Chamomile is known for its relaxing properties, and the flavor is deliciously mild, so that's always a good choice, especially at night. Make your hot beverage more relaxing and spalike by sipping it out of a pretty teacup or mug. Ever wonder why drinking tea is so relaxing? Researchers at University College London say the calming effects may be due to a compound in tea called theanine, which has been shown in lab studies to reduce anxiety. They gave 75 men either tea or a placebo before a stressful test; those who drank the tea had lower poststress responses to the hormone cortisol and also claimed to feel less stressed out.

*Honey.* No tea is complete without a drop of honey. If you don't already have a nice jar of honey at home, get one today. Make sure it is good quality, with nothing added. Raw, organic, unfiltered, US Grade A honey is the best.

*Lemons/oranges/cucumbers.* This may seem a bit over the top, but we promise, this little detail is going to change your life—or at the very least, it will make you smile this weekend. Every great, high-end spa has a pitcher or beverage dispenser filled with water and either lemon, orange, or cucumber slices or some combination of the three. All you need to do is to slice up your favorite flavors, put them in a pitcher of filtered water, and leave the pitcher in the fridge for a few hours. You will not believe how delicious and refreshing plain water tastes all of a sudden—and it helps you relax. When 40 test subjects sniffed various oils and were then given an anxiety-inducing test, those who had smelled orange essential oil were less anxious during the test than the control group, according to a study in Brazil. It's truly amazing. You will want to keep some flavored water in your fridge at all times. This is just one of the small changes you make this weekend that you can incorporate easily into your everyday life.

*Dried fruit and nuts.* It's nice to have a healthy snack around—not just for the spalike ambience but also for your overall health and well-being. Choose dried fruit with no added sugar or preservatives and nuts that are raw, not roasted and/or salted. Leave these in small, pretty dishes or bowls around your home this weekend. Nuts contain many heart-healthy substances: Unsaturated fats, or "good" fats, help lower bad cholesterol levels. Omega-3 fatty acids, also found in many kinds of fish, guard against heart attacks. The fiber in nuts keeps you feeling full longer. And nuts' vitamin E stops the development of plaque in arteries. A bowl of dried fruit and nuts is another small detail that will make you smile—and keep your snacks healthy, too!

*Flowers.* Nothing is prettier, or makes us smile more, than fresh flowers. Seeing and smelling them can change your entire mood. But a fragrant bouquet is more than just pretty and sweet. Research suggests that flowers have both immediate and long-term effects on emotional reactions, mood, social behaviors, and even memory for both guys and gals. A study published in *Evolutionary Psychology* found that when flowers are presented to women, it always elicits a smile, and a woman's positive mood lasts for up to 3 days after she receives the flowers. Treat yourself to beautiful blossoms and place them in vases around your home. (We know you have plenty of vases tucked away!) Get enough flowers so that you can have them in your living room, in your kitchen and dining area, and on your nightstand.

*Eye mask.* Feel the urge to take a leisurely nap? An eye mask can be helpful if you are sensitive to light. It's also an inexpensive way to feel extravagant. Hey, it's your weekend—be fabulous!

*Robe.* No spa experience would be complete without a robe. If you don't have one, you might consider purchasing one this weekend—then it's always available whenever you need a break. Fluffy white terry cloth robes are cozy and soft, but you can also find lighter cotton robes that fall to the knee and are easier to wear around the house. There is nothing more decadent than lounging around in a robe, and when you are doing your spa treatments (hair mask, face mask, etc.), a

> ## TOP 10 FAVE BLOOMS
> 1. Anemones
> 2. Dahlias
> 3. Gardenias
> 4. Hyacinths
> 5. Hydrangeas
> 6. Orchids
> 7. Peonies
> 8. Ranunculus
> 9. Roses
> 10. Tulips

## Jill

*When I pack for a trip, one thing that always makes it into my bag is a Jo Malone travel candle. This brand is my favorite, and I like to take a little bit of my relaxing and cozy home life with me wherever I go. You will never walk into my bedroom and not find mini-roses (from the deli downstairs) and a candle. It is such an inexpensive way to make my space prettier, softer, and more elegant. Setting the mood in my home environment is so important, especially since I live in a big city and have such a hectic life.*

## Dana

*My home is always stocked with candles, tea, honey, some healthy snacks (nuts and dried fruit), lemons, face and body scrub, flowers, and a robe. I love to light a candle at the end of the day just as the sun starts to go down. It is so calming and soothing. The Kai gardenia-scented candles smell delicious, remind me of summer, are made of all-natural ingredients, come in three sizes, and are made of white wax in a clear glass jar so they go with any décor. In the winter, I also love to relax with a cup of tea and honey. My favorite is Yogi tea (lemon ginger flavor) and Dr. Ben Kim's honey—this honey tastes like butterscotch, yum! Arcona face and body scrubs are part of my regular beauty routine. These divine, all-natural products come from an amazing spa in Santa Monica, California. I use these a couple of times a week in the shower. I pick up fresh flowers every week—whatever looks pretty that day: ranunculus, anemones, hyacinths, tulips, hydrangeas, roses, or peonies (my fave). There's nothing better than the smell of fresh flowers when you enter your home. When I lived in Miami, I always kept a pitcher of water with organic lemon slices in my fridge. It was one of my favorite things. (I need to get back into the habit of doing that!)*

robe is the easiest thing to wear, as you don't have to pull anything on or off over your head to shower or bathe.

You should be able to purchase all of the above supplies (except for the robe and sleep mask) at a market like Whole Foods. The robe and sleep mask are easily found at someplace like Bed Bath & Beyond.

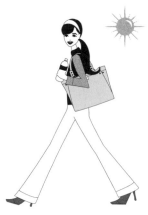

## SATURDAY AFTERNOON

Now that you have your supplies, it's time to "spa-ify" your home. Just by incorporating the following special touches, you will turn your living space into a no-stress zone.

It's fine if you needed your phone while you were out shopping, but now that you are back home, let's return to spa mode. Without all the buzz from the electronics, you may actually enjoy using a "spa voice" as well. That's the quiet, respectful voice you use at the spa when you are calm, relaxed, and not competing with the extraneous noise that comes with daily life.

The afternoon is all yours to spend how you like. We have a suggested schedule based on the typical afternoon spa experience:

Change into your robe.

Put on enjoyable, chill music.

Cut the flower stems and put the blossoms in vases around your home.

Light candles.

Make a cup of tea.

Read a magazine.

Make yourself a healthy lunch—green salad with grilled chicken, fish, or tofu; veggie sandwich on whole grain bread or pita; or gazpacho with some sliced avocado.

If you wish to make your own home-recipe beauty products, you might do that while you are preparing your lunch, so that you are not working in the kitchen all day.

Make a pitcher of lemon, cucumber, or orange water.

Place some healthy snacks (nuts and dried fruit) around.

Have a hot shower and use your face and body scrub to exfoliate all the dead skin cells and bring to the surface fresh, new, brighter skin.

Get back into your robe. *Aah.*

Apply a face mask and a hair mask.

Lounge and read a book while you sit with the masks on. Better yet, soak in the tub *and* read a book at the same time, if you like, while waiting for your masks to do their tricks. Or simply sit with your eyes closed for a peaceful 20 minutes or so.

Shower off the face and hair masks.

Get back into your robe.

Have some hydrating lemon/cucumber/orange water—whichever flavor you made.

Do more lounging and reading.

Put on your eye mask and take a leisurely, decadent afternoon nap.


Now—how do you feel? Have we given you enough to keep you busy today? You'll be amazed how fast the day goes by when you are enjoying yourself! Do any or all of the above: whatever makes you feel most relaxed, pampered, and happy and gives you the sensation of being at a weekend spa escape.

It's amazing what you can do in your own home when you shut off the noise and step out of your daily routine. It doesn't have to cost a fortune to reap the benefits of relaxation. You just need to bring the spa to you.

No stress, no guilt. If it's difficult for you to pamper yourself without feeling guilty, then this weekend is going to be good practice. If you have trouble relaxing because you are thinking of all the other stuff you "should" be doing—household chores, answering e-mails, running errands—then schedule time in the upcoming week to get all of these things done. Literally mark off time slots in your calendar with notes or create a chore list. This way, you can set those worries aside and focus on letting go and relaxing this weekend.

Think of taking care of yourself as a responsibility, too—something that needs to get done, just like all of your other chores. When you take the time to care for yourself, ultimately you will take better care of everyone else around you. Knowing this should alleviate any feelings of being selfish for taking a time-out. It may feel silly to lounge in a robe with a face mask on, but it's important! Taking the time to relax will reenergize you so that you will be up for any activities with your kids.

*Jill* *Aah, downtime. I love it. I don't know about you, but I need to prepare to relax. Yes, I actually have to work to relax. I need everything to be perfect before I can settle in. That means that in addition to having flowers and candles in the house, my bed must be made, my clothes put away, and my things organized. Once that is accomplished, no matter the temperature or time of day, I drink a cup of hot water with lemon. It calms me down and, somehow, mentally tells my body to relax—at least for an hour!*

*Dana* *There's nothing I like better than taking a weekend afternoon to chill. Allowing myself that time, without feeling any pressure to be anywhere, do anything, or see anyone, is the greatest reward I can give myself. I love just lounging in a robe or comfy loungewear, catching up on my magazines or reading a book while surrounded by lit candles, mellow music, and fresh flowers and sipping a cup of tea and honey. Believe it or not, the reading itself (getting through my magazines and reading another book on my list) actually makes me feel productive, even while I am relaxing. It's a win-win!*

Relaxation Makeover          159

How many days do you wake up and wish you didn't have to get dressed and run out the door to work, to carpool, or to what have you? Well, today you get your wish! Feel thankful, not guilty. Just having some peaceful time to yourself will have you ready to take on anything else that comes your way. If you are run ragged on a regular basis (sound familiar?), what kind of attention and care can you give to those around you?

Think also of this weekend as a "free" vacation—you're not at a fancy spa, it just feels like one. We know it's hard to be in your own home and not think about needing more toilet paper or whether there is enough food in the house or if the bills have been paid. Those things will get taken care of. They always do.

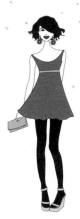

## SATURDAY NIGHT

By now, you should feel like a bowl of Jell-O: totally relaxed and unwound. Enjoy it! You have set aside this weekend for exactly this reason. Stay in your robe and order in take-out food—or if you're in the mood to go out for dinner, that's great, too. Just pick a place with a calm and soothing atmosphere. Surround yourself with people who know what your weekend makeover is all about and who are happy to keep things mellow rather than to paint the town red. And enjoy whatever you end up doing. You're on a mini-break. Remember?

Do you also remember that we told you that a lot of these makeovers would end up overlapping and building on each other? Well, just because you are taking a break from your electronics does not mean you need to stare at the walls all evening. If you chose an evening in (or even when you get home from dinner), take this opportunity to engage in your new activity from Chapter 4. A hobby is meant to be an outlet to relieve stress and nourish the soul.

Practice the piano, paint something, write in your journal, knit, or maybe even bake a few healthy treats for your family to say thanks for supporting you in your efforts to relax this weekend. All of these activities are allowed and actually recommended! Take advantage of this sizeable chunk of time to make some real progress, especially if you are usually only able to squeeze in 15 minutes here and there during a typical week. You could see some real results tonight—maybe you'll finish that scarf, learn a new tune, discover a new recipe, or just finish a thought in your journal or on your blog!

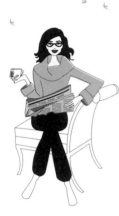

# SUNDAY

Aah, another day at the spa. What to do? Relax and continue to pamper yourself, that's what! Again, you have the day to "spa it" at home. Likely you don't need another face or body scrub, nor do you need another face or hair mask, but you can never get enough of a soothing environment.

Today, continue to leave the cell phone, computer, and TV off. We promise you haven't missed much, if anything! Real life, the news, and everything else will still be there on Monday morning, so don't worry about having been out of the loop for the weekend. Embrace the peace and quiet and the freedom to escape.

Spend more time in your pajamas or robe, even for a little while, to remind yourself that you are off duty. Listen to mellow music, read, make a pot of tea. Take another long, luxurious bath. Light candles and soak. Eat light and healthy today. Make another pitcher of your special water (lemon, cucumber, or orange) for the week.

Recharge your batteries. Anything that you like to do that helps you feel relaxed and rejuvenated is encouraged today. If you are thrilled to be catching up on your reading and the weather is not great, carry on. However, if you are eager to get moving and get outside, take advantage of this day to go for a long walk or

*Jill* I consider driving an "activity," and sometimes I even consider traffic a good thing. The car is one of the few places where I cannot text or read e-mails. But I can listen to the radio—something I rarely get to do. For years, when I lived in Miami, I had a convertible. At the time, I was a sportscaster for CBS and my hours were nuts: anchoring the 6:00 and 11:00 p.m. news. I was in and out at odd times. I used to cherish the ride there and back. It would sometimes take me an hour to get to work with traffic (usually an 18-minute ride), but I loved the trip (most of the time). My ex-boyfriend smoked cigars a lot. We used to take long drives; he would smoke his cigar, and we would listen to music and laugh. I'm relaxed just thinking about it. (For the record, I do not smoke cigars, but I do like the aroma!) I have learned not to be bothered by traffic but rather to relish the time away from my other responsibilities.

*Dana* One of my favorite things to do when I lived in LA was to jump in my car, open the windows, blast the music, and drive out to Malibu. Sometimes when I got out there, I wouldn't even step out of the car! I just wanted to see and smell the ocean, and I loved the drive itself. This was especially important when I returned from a visit to New York City. I would literally go home, drop my suitcase, change clothes, and hop in the car for a drive. It didn't matter that I had just flown 6 hours on a plane. I craved the fresh ocean air and the view.

hike or take a yoga class. If the weather allows, get outside and lie in the sun. Feel the warmth on your face (don't forget to wear SPF!) and let the sun melt your muscles into deep relaxation.

Are you in the mood for more pampering? Treat yourself to a massage, a facial, a manicure/pedicure, or even a hair blowout. We will put money on the fact that these are rare occurrences in your daily life, and that generally even when you do stop for a quick pedicure, you are still multitasking at the time—answering calls and e-mails while your toenails are being polished or, even worse, juggling your phone and typing with one finger while the other hand's nails are being polished. Sound familiar?

Take the time today to do something you normally wouldn't do or that you would otherwise rush through. Have brunch with a girlfriend—with no phones on the table! Browse through your favorite bookstore. Go to a matinee movie all by yourself—see something your husband would never agree to—and escape into the dark theater. Treat yourself to something new for your wardrobe (only if it's a perfect 10, of course!)

If driving doesn't stress you and you want to get out of town, hop in the car, open the windows, put on your favorite music, and take a drive to the country or the beach or along any scenic road that makes you feel like you're escaping for a bit.

Now that you have experienced what it's like to really indulge and relax, let's make a plan to incorporate aspects of this weekend into your daily life.

- Promise yourself that you will keep your house stocked with candles, tea, honey, healthy snacks, and lemon-, cucumber-, and/or orange-flavored water. (The latter should be a no-brainer, since you can just add the ingredients to your grocery list when you run out.)

- Remember to light candles every evening when you are home to soften the mood and give your home a nice, relaxing glow.

- Make yourself a cup of tea with honey after dinner to sip slowly and help you unwind from the day.

- Promise yourself that you will treat yourself (and your home) to fresh flowers every week.

- If you have kept up with your beauty makeover, you have already set aside the time for a face scrub and mask on Sunday evening (or whichever night you chose), so add to that regimen the hair mask and a nice hot bath. Wash it all off and do a body scrub at the same time.

- Make a pact with yourself for a certain amount of electronic gadget–free time every week. Commit to shutting off your phone, computer, and TV and listening to peaceful music instead. Decide what works for you. Maybe everything gets shut off after a certain hour every evening. Maybe it's a few nights a week that you refrain, or maybe it is one day per weekend, or some combination of the above.

- Remind yourself that it's okay—even better than okay; it's well deserved— that you allow yourself some lounge time in your robe or favorite pajamas. Schedule that into your weekend or evening routine.

- And even better—promise yourself that you will put on your eye mask, take a nap when you need one, and not feel the slightest bit guilty about it. We are not talking about initiating a daily nap, but on a lazy Saturday or Sunday afternoon, you are entitled!

- Promise yourself that you will take the time to read a book or your favorite magazines instead of reading you need to do for work or watching TV. If you have kept up with your clutter makeover (see Chapter 8), you have been keeping current with your periodicals. If reading was one of the activities you chose in the brain makeover (see Chapter 5), then see—you are already incorporating this in your repertoire, and you don't need to set aside extra time.

- Do something that relieves your stress at least once a month—head outside, take a hike, change your scenery, get out of the city or out of town for a few hours, indulge in a massage, jump in the ocean, browse or shop for things that are not considered "errands" (like books or a new purse or pair of shoes), have lunch with a friend. Do all of these things without your cell phone!

Congrats on turning your home into a successful home spa! We know it was a lot to ask to completely shut off for the weekend, but you did it! We hope (and are pretty sure) you feel relaxed, refreshed, and rejuvenated—like a brand-new you. Enjoy the rest of Sunday night before you dive back into the workweek. Sleep well—you're ready to get back in the game tomorrow with a whole new outlook and your batteries completely recharged.

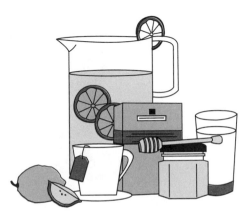

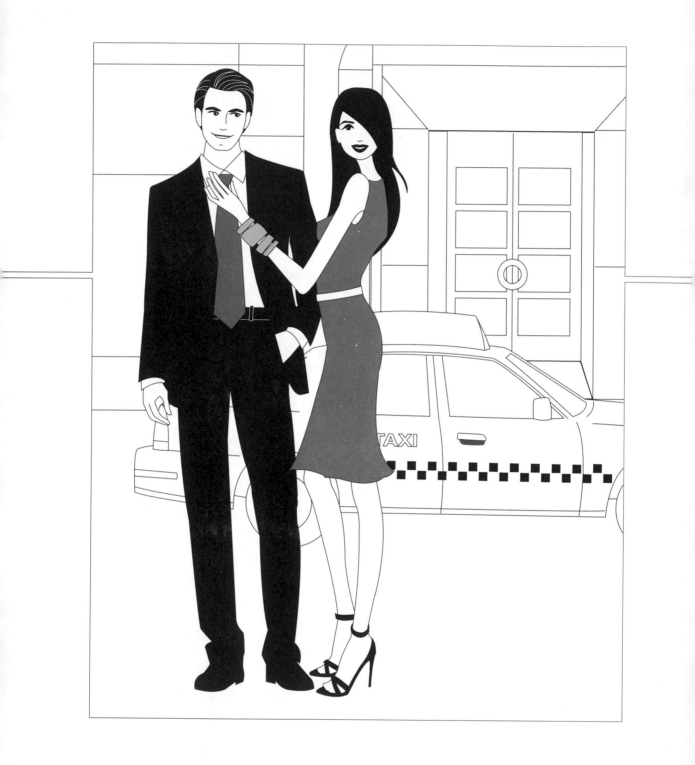

# Chapter Ten
# Relationship Makeover

Has your relationship lost the spark it once had? Have you lost sight of what attracted you to your partner in the first place? Are your lives so busy with work, kids, and, well, life that you don't get quality time with your boyfriend, partner, or spouse anymore? You're not alone. One survey conducted by Cove Haven Entertainment Resorts found that nearly half of respondents had not been on vacation with just their partner within the past year, while more than half hadn't even been out for a romantic dinner in at least 6 months.

The phenomenon of growing apart over time because of life's pressures and distractions happens all too frequently, and most people think it's just "the way it is" after you've been with someone for a while. Well, we are here to tell you that it doesn't have to be this way. In fact, it should *not* be this way. With a bit of work and dedication to getting your relationship back on track, you will be on the road to a more functional, more rewarding, and more fulfilling relationship—in just one weekend. Doesn't that sound much better than chalking up faded passion to age, time, or whatever other excuse you can come up with? We thought so!

This weekend, you will get to know and fall in love with your partner all over again. But first, he needs to be available! Make sure he knows in advance that you want to spend the weekend together. If you have kids, preschedule them to be out of the house—at the grandparents' or with friends—because you need to focus this weekend on just each other.

Start with a commitment to your relationship and the desire to make it the best it can be. You are devoting a weekend to each other, so jump in with both feet and your whole heart. You'll do everything from revamping his look (if he needs an update and he's game!) to spending serious quality time together. Are you ready to get started?

## ☾ FRIDAY NIGHT

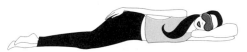

We hope you've both set this weekend aside to spend real time together, improve your relationship, and have fun. We're also hoping that your partner is game to humor you in all that you ask of him this weekend.

**Just the two of you.** Tonight, have dinner together. Stay in or go out. Either choice is fine, just as long as there are no distractions—work, kids, e-mails, cell phones, etc. Talk about what activities you want to do this weekend and what you hope to accomplish. Make sure he understands that this weekend is all about making your lives better together (even as you oh-so-kindly clean out his closet tomorrow morning!). Get him, and yourself, excited to bond and enjoy each other's company.

Explain to him (in the nicest way possible) that you'd like to spend the day tomorrow stepping up his wardrobe game. Then plan a real "date night" for Saturday evening. And let him know that on Sunday, you want to work out together, eat together, relax together, and enjoy additional special time together.

Commit to going to bed together at the same time for the next 3 nights (yes, Sunday night is still part of the weekend). Plan to start your mornings together, too. Spend extra time in bed rekindling the intimacy that gets lost in your all-too-busy lives. There is nothing and no one but the two of you this weekend. Laugh, have sex, cuddle, and remember what drew you to your beloved in the first place. Practice having fun in your relationship again! In a survey published by North Carolina State University, when couples were asked what would improve their relationship, 62 percent listed spending more time together. Researcher John Gottman says that couples who spend 5 hours a week together maintain successful relationships. Once you have your partner's time, spend some of it talking. Forty percent of those who completed the survey said communication was the most successful element in their relationship.

Sleep well together!

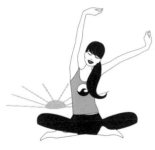

## SATURDAY MORNING

Part of being attracted to your mate is his appearance, which reflects his personality and style. You were drawn to each other to begin with, so he couldn't have been a disaster in the style department—unless, of course, you are that girl who said to yourself, "No big deal, I can change him." Hmm, how did that work out for you?

Chances are good that he doesn't need a whole new look, but he just needs to get back to being a "10" in your eyes. Let's start by asking the same questions you applied to your closet—this time, you'll be the kind, honest, loving friend for him.

You have already (we hope) gone through your wardrobe and done a makeover on your own closet, so you should know exactly what to do with your partner's closet. (If you need a reference, see Chapter 7 for all of the guidelines on what to keep, what to toss, and where to get rid of the items you are not keeping.)

A quick refresher of the eight wardrobe criteria questions—plus one more question directed to you:

1. Is the garment in perfect condition—no holes, no pills, and no stains?

2. Does it represent his personality—meaning does he look like him when he wears it?

3. Does it fit his lifestyle—meaning does he have occasion to wear it?

4. Is it age appropriate?

5. Is it location/climate appropriate?

6. Does he wear or has he ever actually worn it?

7. Does it fit in with his personal style?

8. Does it fit and flatter his frame perfectly?

9. And most important, do *you* like it on him?

**Be honest, yet realistic.** The truth is, while the answer to the first eight questions might be yes, the last one could be no. If this is the case, you might sweetly explain why that particular look just doesn't turn you on—or you might decide to move on. The process is a give-and-take, and you'll have to compromise (surely he keeps opinions to himself about some of the things you wear!). People should have the right to wear what they like and express themselves as they see fit. That said, there is a gentle way to encourage him to wear things you find attractive. You may never be able to throw away his college sweatshirt, but you can certainly show him how much more alluring you find him in that sharp sports coat!

If you have been keeping mental notes about certain garments (such as thoughts of secretly dumping them), start with those pieces. Be honest about what you like and what you don't—but stay positive. At the same time that you are walking him through the items you don't like, encourage him by pointing out your favorite pieces and the clothing you truly love on him. This way, you can carefully guide him toward dressing in clothing that pleases you and that is already part of his repertoire.

Believe it or not, men can be more insecure about the way they dress and how they look than women! It's not considered "manly" if a guy cares about how he looks, so oftentimes men don't pay much attention, or they are afraid to ask for

*Jill* *I have had three serious relationships in my life. No offense to any of my exes reading this, but none of them were major fashion statements. I have learned to pick my battles. I will never press a man to wear something he is not comfortable in. However, I do think it is important to always be appropriately dressed. If an event calls for black tie, a man should be dressed accordingly. If a dinner or party is at someone's home, a sloppy T-shirt is not going to cut it. My father is a very casual man. He doesn't like getting dressed up, so I rarely pick restaurants or venues where he can't wear a polo shirt and his boat shoes. Sometimes, you just have to know your audience.*

*Dana* *The number-one question men ask me when they find out I am a fashion stylist is, "How do I look?" And the next question is, "Is my outfit okay?" It's truly amazing. These are usually total strangers! I can be at a party, and as soon as the topic of my work comes up, that's the first thing out of their mouths. Mind you, women never ask! I have women friends who will ask what to wear before an event, or ask for help shopping, etc., but never has a woman I just met ever asked me, "How do I look?" Men really don't know, and they so desperately want and need the reassurance that they are on the right track. They are happy to hear me tell them that they look totally appropriate and they did a great job dressing themselves. Seriously, you should see the smiles of relief and pride!*

help. Here is your opportunity. Flattery will get you everywhere!

Go through his closet, piece by piece. If you get to an item that you don't like and that he agrees to part with, you can move along. If there is an item you both want to keep, run through the first eight criteria questions to determine if it is a 10 and should stay in his wardrobe.

Remember, men gain and lose weight, just like women do. Men change careers, move to different climates, and age out of certain styles. They hang on to items that are no longer in perfect condition. And they, too, make bad wardrobe purchases and end up with things that still have the price tags on! When you are done clearing out the clothing items you never want to see again, neatly organize the remaining "keep" items so that he has a functional closet, same as you.

Take stock of what remains in his wardrobe. You agree that these are all pieces you both like and that you would like to see him in all of the time. Correct? Okay, great. Let's look to fill in the gaps with similar items and possibly some new options. It is more than likely that you just completed a massive cleanout. This afternoon, you have the opportunity to fill out his wardrobe so that he has a good number of choices in his rotation.

Before we get ahead of ourselves, though, you need to figure out exactly what you want to add to his wardrobe. If he already owns really great pieces and you'd like to purchase more of the same, fantastic. If there are wardrobe looks you'd like him to try, ease him into the idea by showing him pictures in a magazine, or online, of some of your fave men's styles.

Do you feel yourself bonding with your partner already? We hope you had many laughs when going through his closet. And we hope he was laughing with you! That's really the point of this exercise. Of course, we want you to have a hot, sexy, perfect-10 man, but he is already that—you chose him! What you and he are gaining from this activity is a reminder that he is your perfect guy, a renewal of his self-esteem, and a resurgence of your attraction to each other—along with a good, strong dose of quality time.

Take a break—together. Have lunch, either at home or at a restaurant you agree on, and get ready for more fun and bonding this afternoon.

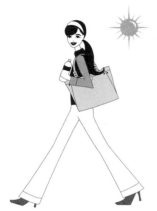

# SATURDAY AFTERNOON

Okay, the hard part (and the dirty work) of the weekend is over. From here on out, it should be smooth sailing. (We hope!) After lunch, you'll hit the stores and get him some new duds. You've already discussed, and decided together, how you'd like to see him dress. Now it's just a matter of shopping.

**Shop smart.** We know: Not everyone loves to shop—this goes for men and women alike. So pick your venues wisely. Take into account what you are looking to buy, where you will find the most variety to choose from, and which stores will give you the most bang for your buck (if that is a concern). Rome wasn't built in a day, and your man's wardrobe won't be, either. Maximize your time so you don't burn out.

Never buy anything because you feel pressured. You know what it's like to shop when you are in dire need of a dress or an outfit for a specific event occurring *that night*. You run around, like a chicken with its head cut off, to a ton of stores, spending way too much money on pieces that aren't right, that you don't need, and that you'll never wear again. Sound about right? Enough said.

Same is true for men. A wardrobe is best built gradually. It should be a collection of quality, perfect-10 pieces that are accumulated over time. Remember, the new clothing you purchase (today and always) must meet the same criteria that his clothing had to meet this morning to justify remaining in the closet.

**Build stylish sex appeal together.** This is going to be a fun afternoon that's all about him (or so he thinks!). If this ends up being an enjoyable activity for both of you, perhaps you can incorporate shopping excursions into your lives—not every weekend, of course. But when the seasons change, or he has a special event or trip coming up and would like some new things, take him shopping. Or maybe when you are out shopping, you can pick up some pieces for him on occasion. Or maybe, just maybe, after today he will feel so much more confident with his style and what he is shopping for that he can handle it all on his own. Sometimes all people need is a push in the right direction!

Today, let's look to purchase new items that are on par with his revamped and upgraded style. This is your opportunity to have him try on pieces that he wouldn't necessarily pick out on his own, so take advantage of this moment to help him see how great he looks in something he might never have considered wearing before. Hint: Sometimes they just need to see it on. (This is true of women, too, by the way!) It can be that easy to help him look and feel confident and sexy. It's so rare that the man gets to be the center of attention on shopping excursions. (Ladies, you are going to have to refrain from having a wandering eye; keep it focused on the men's department this afternoon!) Today, it is all about him.

Spend as much time shopping this afternoon as you are both comfortable with. Stop *before* anyone gets tired or cranky. If you make a few key purchases that look and fit great, and that you both love, consider yourselves successful and call it a day. You've worked hard, and you still want to have energy for your date tonight!

*Jill* *Pick your battles. If you find a brand that fits well and that your partner likes, buy a few of the same items in different colors or patterns. I know very few men who like to spend the day shopping, so take that into account if your man is not one of them, and keep the excursion short and sweet.*

*Dana* *I shop for a living, and even I reach my limit. There have been times that I have been in one store, or the mall, for so many hours on end that I can feel myself about to lose it and I just have to get out. When I feel like this, I am no longer productive, I can't focus, and I physically need to leave. It's definitely better to stop shopping way before you get to this point!*

Well done! Your feet are probably tired, so why don't the two of you take an afternoon siesta together before you get ready for your Saturday night out? It's your weekend to devote to each other—so if you both just want to nap, crawl into bed together. You never know what may happen, and there's nothing around to distract you or grab your attention! Focus on enjoying some quiet time together.

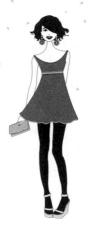

# SATURDAY NIGHT

It's Saturday night—date night. Maybe you haven't experienced this in a while? That's okay. We're pretty sure you'll remember what it's like to get dressed up, put on some makeup, and actually leave the house for a fun night out.

Now, when we say "fun," we are leaving the interpretation of that word up to you. We're not implying that you need to go crazy and stay out till 3:00 in the morning just because the kids are away! However, if that is "fun" to you, by all means, go for it!

**Shake things up.** Select an activity that you both love but haven't done in a while. If you usually go out for dinner and a movie, try bowling or dancing. If you both love music or theater, check out a concert or a show or a jazz club. Pick something that will bring back happy memories, or choose something that you have been meaning to do but just never got around to. If you don't often go out, something as simple as dinner and a movie (or a long evening stroll) will feel magical.

The point of this evening, and this whole weekend, is to spend more quality time with your man, learn how to make your relationship a priority, and fall in love all over again. Today was a great start. He now has some

> ## TOP **10** DATE NIGHT IDEAS
> 1. Art exhibit
> 2. Bowling
> 3. Concert
> 4. Dancing
> 5. Moonlight stroll
> 6. Movie
> 7. Romantic dinner
> 8. Sporting event
> 9. Stargazing
> 10. Theater

fabulous new pieces in his wardrobe from which to put together an outfit for tonight. You both should look hot tonight for your date and for each other. Tell him how handsome he looks. Encourage him to please you all the time, and do the same for him. Put on your go-to evening makeup look that you learned in Chapter 3, or try out a more daring, sexy look for this evening. It takes just a little bit of effort to look great rather than okay, and you know how, so do it!

When you look great, you feel great. This goes for men too. Self-confidence stems from feeling good. We all know how much more confidence we exude when we know we look hot. And confidence is just about the sexiest quality there is.

It's so easy to fall into a rut. Especially when we've been with the same partner for years, we forget how important it is to keep the relationship alive and interesting. Most often, people complain that their long-term relationship has turned into a partnership rather than a romantic relationship. And while the day-to-day routine definitely becomes part of the relationship equation, and the mortgage and kids naturally take priority, everyone deserves romance, too! A little tweak to the wardrobe (and, if you want to take it a step further, grooming) and committing to spend real quality time together are sometimes all it takes to jump-start the passion back in your relationship and remind you what attracted you to this person in the first place.

**Share the moment.** Whatever you decide to do tonight, be present. No phones, no e-mails, no texting. Your priority, and your focus, is your partner and your relationship. Nothing else matters right now. (If you have already done the home spa makeover in Chapter 9, you will be familiar and comfortable with the

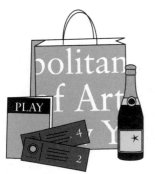

process of shutting off from the outside world for a bit.) Ask him to be present, too.

Talk to each other, find out what's really going on with each other, and make plans for your future. This is a time-out for both of you. Take advantage of this weekend bubble you are creating to make sure you are both happy and fulfilled and to discuss how to get there, if your relationship has weak spots. Taking this time to recommit to each other is a great place to start.

*Jill* *I once dated a younger man—it didn't last long, but he did teach me one thing. We were going out on a Saturday night, and he asked me not to bring my phone. He pointed out that I am constantly checking it and told me that I am not the President of the United States and nothing is so pressing that I can't have a date night without interruption. Although we weren't right for each other, because of him, I will never carry my BlackBerry on a date again. Sounds obvious, but it was something I needed to learn. Leave it to the (much) younger guy to make me aware of it!*

*Dana* *There is nothing better (to me) than just holding hands and going for a walk with my man. I don't care about big fancy dinners or loud clubs. Of course, going out dancing is fun every once in a while, but being able to talk and simply spend quality alone time is my favorite. Ideally, this walk would be on a secluded beach somewhere in really warm weather!*

Most of all, tonight simply enjoy and remember what it is like to have fun!

When you get home, continue the date. No running to the computer, checking e-mails, texting, or anything of the sort. Make sure you end the night together. No watching TV in separate rooms or going to bed at different times. You made a promise at the beginning of the weekend to go to bed together every night. We have a feeling after your hot date, you will want to anyway!

# SUNDAY

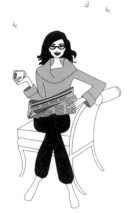

When you wake up, linger in bed together. If this opportunity or occurrence is rare, relish it. Hang out, curl up, have sex, or all of the above. Remember when you first started spending time at each other's places and there was nowhere else you needed or wanted to be? That's what we want you to feel now. Back before the kids, before the heavy responsibilities: when nothing was more important than being with the person you were madly in love with. Somehow time seemed slower then, or there wasn't as much on the to-do list, or, well, maybe the to-do list just wasn't a priority.

**Slow it down.** This morning, make each other the priority, not your errands. Think about how you used to spend your weekend mornings together and pretend you were back in one of your old haunts. Did you eat breakfast in bed, lounge around reading the paper, or have long talks about your future? Do whatever you both enjoyed together.

All those joint plans for the future—have they happened? Take time now to regroup on what you both want to work toward—old plans and dreams that may not have come to fruition and new plans and dreams that you may not have talked about yet. Working together toward your joint future stimulates and supports your relationship.

Today is another chance to spend time together. Figure out what you both would like to do and how to spend it. Yesterday, you were hard at work closet cleaning and on a shopping mission. Today, reward yourself with relaxing activities. Go for a walk, bike ride, or hike—together. Take an exercise class or go to the gym—together. Afterward, indulge in a delicious yet healthy brunch (again, with no phones!).

If you choose to lounge at home, spend time in the same room. Curl up and read the paper together or watch a movie together or both. Have a cozy evening in, cook a meal together, and share a bottle of wine.

**Keep the weekend going.** Talk about ways that you can incorporate facets of this weekend into your everyday lives. We know it gets superhectic with work, kids, and every other distraction, but just as you have made time for other makeovers, make time for this one, too. It may be the most important commitment you make.

Discuss what's realistic for a regular date night. Choose new and exciting things to do occasionally, rather than trying to go out all the time. Doing a new activity together will rekindle the emotions you felt when you first started dating. Make sure you have date night at least twice a month. Once a week is ideal, if you can swing a babysitter. Choose a night that works for both of you. It can be on the weekend or during the week, or it can vary according to other commitments. Just make sure you put something in the books and that you make it happen.

On date night, dress up for each other. This doesn't mean black-tie dressy. What it does mean is that you strive to look like a 10 for your mate and for yourself, and he should do the same. Compliment him often. Make him feel confident and sexy. Ask him to do the same for you.

**Sleep together.** Make a pact that you will go to sleep together every night that you are able to. We know not everyone's schedules are always in sync with work, kids, and what have you, but if you can commit to at least 1 night a week (or both weekend nights) to do this, it will be a great start. Remember, it only takes 21 days to form or break a habit. Get back in the habit of shared bedtime. It is crucial to have a connection at the end of your busy day, and it's not always about sex—just the connection.

Remember to shut off your phones when you are spending quality time together. No one else (besides your kids, of course) is more important. Make time together count.

What a weekend! You dug in and did serious work on your man and your relationship. What a great reminder of why you got into this relationship in the first place! Now, provided that you keep it up (and we know that you will), you can sit back and reap the rewards. Great job, you two!

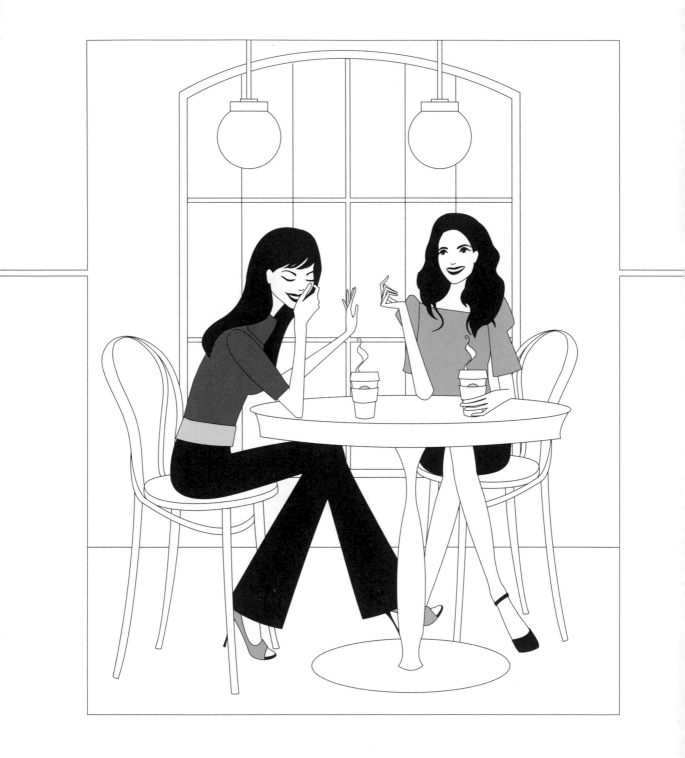

# *Chapter Eleven*
# Friendship Makeover

Do you feel like it's been ages since you've caught up with your best friends? Has your social circle noticeably shrunk in recent years? Is the number of people on your "must call" list so long that you don't even know where to begin and sometimes find it easier to avoid callbacks altogether?

We hear you. Somehow life keeps getting busier and faster, and even the best-laid plans can get sidelined.

There's nothing worse than running into a friend with whom you have long been MIA and trying to come up with a lame excuse for your behavior. It doesn't feel good for the friend, and it doesn't feel good for you, either! This weekend, you will change all that. No more feeling bad or guilty because you owe someone a phone call, an e-mail, or even just a text. If you don't have time for the most basic forms of contact, we can only wonder how you ever make time to see anyone outside of work and your immediate family. Or do you?

We're not entirely sure that you *don't* have the time. Perhaps you have been so overwhelmed with life that you don't know where or how to reconnect. (Hopefully, if you've been following this book, things in your life are more under control!)

Maintaining friendships is important—and not just for your social life. It's actually good for your health. A 10-year Australian study found that older people with a large circle of friends were 22 percent less likely to die during the study period than those with fewer friends. And in 2011, Harvard researchers reported that strong social ties could promote brain health as we age.

This is why you need a break, a time-out, to get your social life back under control. This weekend, you are going to reevaluate your friendships and take responsibility for how you've been neglecting them (however innocently it all started). Over the next couple of days, you'll reconnect with the people you have been missing and plan a strategy to stay on top of relationships so you don't fall out of touch again.

The project for this weekend is not labor intensive, but it requires that you prioritize and devote time to handling your personal affairs rather than whatever other business or activities normally take up all of your time. Ready to connect?

## ☾ FRIDAY NIGHT

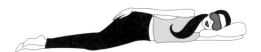

When you want to get something under control but you are overwhelmed and don't know where to begin, the first thing to do is make a list.

Have dinner, think about the situation, and then sit down by yourself for half an hour or so with a cup of tea, a pad and pen, and your contact list or address book. Leave the TV off so you don't get distracted or sidetracked. Start making a list of friends you want to reconnect with.

**List your loved ones.** If you have been neglecting your nearest and dearest, write their names down first. Next, go through your phone and look at the call log, the text messages, and the e-mails. Write down the names of anyone who you have not responded to, know that it's your turn to get in touch with, or just really want to see. When you are done with that, take a look through all of your contacts. There are likely people who have so fallen by the wayside that no text message or missed call is still on record in your phone.

Feels good just to know that you are on the road to reconnecting with the important people in your life, doesn't it? There's nothing like a good catch-up with a longtime dear friend whom you (and probably, she, too) have been too busy to see or speak with.

But what about those people who were once a big part of your life but don't fit anymore? Good question. This weekend is for you to think about who is important to you and who you want to have in your life. You have spent many other weekends making over your home, your body, and your mind. This weekend is no different. Take the time to declutter your social life, and it will also feel more balanced and harmonious.

We're not saying that you dump everyone you don't have time for. What we are saying is to find ways to make time for the friends you want to retain. Go through your list and highlight the people you definitely need to stay in touch with. Maybe you want to keep everyone—that's great! Maybe you hold on to some and let others go—that's fine, too. Sometimes people grow apart, move away, and find different paths and interests. Nothing wrong with that. It's okay to appreciate people for who they were to you at one time in your life, even if they don't fit anymore.

You can even go a little further to break down your list into categories:

**People you want to see weekly (or besties).** These are the people who (outside of your immediate family) are most important to you. So even if your days are superbusy, you want to make sure these people have a weekly time slot. Up to you how many people are on this list and how you schedule them in, but you definitely want to make sure these plans happen. It can be anything from a standing coffee date, to an exercise class and a juice, to a night out on the town.

**People you want to speak to monthly (or close friends).** These are people who you really enjoy, but might not be your nearest and dearest. Or, possibly, they are very close to you, but they don't live nearby, or for whatever reason your

## Jill

I went to college at the University of Michigan, and there were eight of us who were the closest of friends. We used to make bets as to who was going to get married first, have kids first, and move away from home. We knew each other inside and out. But after we graduated, as every year passed, the friendships started to drift away. There was a 10-year chunk of time that I really did not keep in touch with the girls who basically had helped mold me into who I am now. Writing this book prompted me to reach out to most of the clan. It was emotional to meet their kids and husbands. We had always spoken about how our lives would turn out, so it was funny to see how they actually played out. I feel much better that we reconnected. It was like a part of me had been missing.

## Dana

When I was growing up, I went to school with the same friends from kindergarten through high school. There was never much effort needed to stay in touch, because I saw everyone almost every day. After I graduated, I moved and have since lived in three different cities. It takes an effort to stay in touch with everyone I am close to, especially when they don't live in the same city—Jill, Alyssa, and Amy live in New York City, Mary Jean and Lizzie are in Los Angeles, and Tiffany is in Miami. And now that a lot of my friends have families and kids, there is a whole other dimension to trying to maintain closeness. Sometimes the onus of the phone call, text, or e-mail falls on me (because I travel so much). But with the people I am closest to, I would never stand on ceremony. I am always glad I made the effort.

schedules really don't mesh so a weekly date is tough to arrange. You don't want to lose track of these friends. If you can see them even a few times a year, great, but keeping in close contact with a catch-up phone session monthly will ensure that you keep them in your life in a substantial way. And, hey, you never know—people move, schedules change, and one day you may be back to weekly plans with this friend!

**People you don't want to lose contact with (or acquaintances).** And then, of course, there are the people in your life who would be considered acquaintances. This is usually the largest group, but with the least amount of maintenance. Keeping these relationships intact can be as simple as liking their status update on Facebook, sending a periodic email, or reaching out during the holiday season with a card.

This weekend, however, we will concentrate on the friends you want to keep but may have been neglecting. Make sure your list is complete. We'll start reconnecting in the morning. By the way, if you are enjoying the quiet time and want to reach out and call someone this evening for a long overdue chat, by all means, please do!

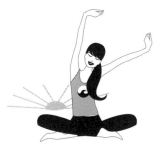

# SATURDAY MORNING

Are you excited to get started? To reconnect? Relax, have breakfast, and then get cozy with your computer and your phone!

This morning is all about digging yourself out of the hole. You are done with the excuses and the guilt. Now, log in to your personal e-mail account and, beginning with the oldest e-mail in your in-box, start responding.

**Be honest.** You don't have to make up crazy stories about why you have been out of touch. (No one believes those anyway.) Just apologize for having been out of touch and explain how you'd like to reconnect. Tell your friend that you would like either to catch up properly over the phone (if she lives far away) or to make a date to see her in person. Of course, you can write a bit about what's going on in

*Jill* *Because of the nature of my business, I get hundreds of e-mails a day. Most are work related, some are from friends, and others are random e-mails (that we all get). I used to let them pile up and then assign days where I would go through everything and feel totally overwhelmed. I have a new rule now. At the end of every day, I go through my e-mail: erase, sort, and organize. I feel so much lighter now. I make the effort to respond to every e-mail. If people take the time to e-mail me, they deserve a response.*

*Dana* *I always try to respond to my friends' e-mails and texts in a timely manner—usually the same day or, at the very least, the next. If I'm having a crazy busy workday, I will leave the personal messages until the end of the day, when I have time to sit down and respond properly— answering all questions asked, engaging with my own questions, and oftentimes making plans to see friends. I feel much better when I don't leave anything untended in my life—including my friendships.*

your world in the e-mail and ask how she is, but if you want to maintain a close friendship, nothing beats a call or an actual visit.

You are taking the time this weekend to nurture the relationships you care about and want to maintain and grow. If you sincerely don't care—or have simply lost interest—with one or some of the people in your in-box, don't pretend to make plans or call and then never do. Let those go, and move on to the people who made your list last night.

Keep going until you have written to all of the people you owe e-mails. Next, go through your phone and respond to the text messages that you have been too busy to answer. There is certainly less to say via text than via e-mail, so these should be pretty easy for you to whip through. Again, be truthful. No more excuses, and no more pretending with people you are never going to make the effort to spend time with.

**Make social media work for you.** Facebook is a completely acceptable place to prune your friend list and stay in touch with those you don't want to lose contact with. You can change your privacy settings to add people to a "limited profile," which allows them to see only your basic info. And it's not a crime to "defriend" someone! According to a Pew Research Center survey of people who use social networking sites, 63 percent have deleted people from their friends lists, up from 56 percent in 2009. The same survey reported that the average number of Facebook friends is 229. If you have over 1,000 "friends," maybe it's time to rethink how you really know all of these people.

Facebook, Twitter, and other social media sites are all well and good for what they are, and they definitely serve a purpose. But for maintaining and nurturing relationships, social sites don't cut it. Want to reconnect with someone from high school, just for the fun of it? Facebook is fine for that. You can use social media to get your new product or business off the ground through your friends and acquaintances, too. It's even fine to check Facebook for birthday reminders if you don't want to keep those dates in your calendar. But if you want to consider someone a close friend, communicating through Facebook or Twitter alone is not enough. It doesn't feel special hearing about a friend's engagement or new baby—along with countless others. It's fine to post pictures and share fun moments online, but make sure you share important news personally with the people closest to you before you post it.

Great job this morning. You should feel lighter already. You have made a decision about the people you want in your life and have started reclaiming those valuable friendships. Take a little break. This afternoon, we take the next step.

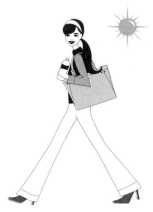

# SATURDAY AFTERNOON

This morning, you took your first step toward getting your friendships back on track and climbing out of the bubble of your own chaotic daily life. Everybody is so busy these days, we seem to forget how important and how nice it is to spend time with someone in person.

We can all make the time. It's just a matter of planning. If you put a date down in your calendar and *commit* to the plan, it will happen—and most often, you'll feel great after a fun night out or coffee date. What happens too frequently is that both parties casually say, "Oh, we'll get together next week sometime," but if there is no solid plan in place, the meeting never comes to fruition.

This afternoon, you are going to remedy that. You will take the initiative and make solid plans. Even with your work, kids, and other commitments, there is time in your month, if not in each week, to squeeze in a lunch, a coffee, a drink, or a dinner with the important people in your life. Don't underestimate how crucial female relationships are in your life and how much you count on your friends' support, their advice, and mostly their ear.

If you've been following along with the previous makeovers, you've found the time to successfully incorporate your workout, your hobby, your extracurricular class (or other learning), your spa moments, and your man into your hectic life. Now it's time to add in one more (very important) thing—your girlfriends.

**Make a date.** Break out your calendar, whether you use a paper date book or track your schedule on your computer or smartphone, and look for empty slots of

## 13 FUN FRIEND DATE ACTIVITIES

1. Beach day
2. Brunch
3. Coffee/tea/juice
4. Concert
5. Day road trip
6. Dinner
7. Drinks
8. Farmers' market
9. Flea market
10. Hike/long walk
11. Museum/art gallery
12. Shopping
13. Theater

## Jill

*I have lost relationships because of text and e-mail. Things get misconstrued, you can't read someone's tone, and the conversations are disjointed. I once dated a guy who told me that if you have something to say, pick up the phone. He mistook an e-mail from me as rude when I was just trying to be funny—and one thing I would never be is rude! If you want to say something right, dial someone's digits! When I first moved to Miami, I met Melissa, and we became inseparable. We've been through breakups, makeups, move-outs, a wedding, and (hopefully soon!) children. Melissa makes sure we see each other once a month. A few years later, while I was still living in Florida, I met my girlfriend Lyndsey and her beautiful family Matt, Olivia, and Jaxson. She is the consummate mother and wife, and she has taught me so much about love and life. I am grateful to have them in my life . . . friends make you stronger and better.*

## Dana

*I travel a lot to see my family and friends, and I get out of the city as often as I can. Every time I come back, even if I've been gone for only the weekend, I go through my phone and reach out to my friends to make plans for the upcoming week or two. It's always nice, especially after being away (or going through a busy work period), to reconnect. Sometimes, those plans don't happen right away, but I never want to let too much time pass without keeping up with the people who are important to me. I have a couple of close friends who also love to do yoga. We even love the same teacher—Elena Brower at Virayoga in New York. Fortunately, I am able to coordinate with Daniela or Gabriela for a yoga date almost weekly, and then we go for lunch or a juice. We are able to catch up and get our workout in—the best of both worlds!*

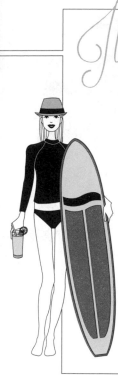

*Jill* *Dana is one of my best friends and we know each other's "stuff" really well. We have both been through love, pain, and growth. Of course, there are topics (the wrong guy) we are both sick of hearing from about each other (and ourselves!), but we always share. I know when I bring up a certain someone, she may roll her eyes, but I know she will listen. This is true for both of us. You have to be there for your friends to listen to the good news and the news you wish would just go away!*

*Dana* *I am still very close with my friends from high school. Three of us meet for lunch about once a month or once every other month. Erica is married with two kids, lives in Brooklyn, and works in Harlem. Stephanie is married with three kids, lives in Westchester, and works in Midtown 2 days a week. I am single and live and work in Chelsea. Even with our three schedules and locations, we figure out a way to coordinate and make it work. It takes a little planning and effort, and it is totally worth it.*

time that you can fill with dates with friends. Perhaps you have Wednesday lunches free, or Thursday after work you can fit in drinks, or Monday afternoon you have time for coffee, or twice a month, your husband won't mind feeding the kids and you can make a dinner date.

It doesn't even have to be the same time slot every week. Take account of where you can realistically fit in a date. And the event doesn't have to revolve around food or drinks. Schedule a workout or running session with your friend, if you're both interested (talk about killing two birds with one stone!). A walk in the park can also be a refreshing change of pace, or even doing chores together—you can turn a typical day at the market into a fun, gossip-filled stroll as you're each stocking your kitchen with delicious, healthy options!

This morning, when you responded to all of the e-mails and texts, you may have mentioned making plans to see certain people. Now that you have your calendar in front of you, reach out again with a few time slot choices so that you can commit to concrete plans. Work your way down the list, either in order of importance or in order of whom you haven't seen the longest.

You can choose to e-mail, text, or, better yet, call your friends to make plans. Depending on how long your list is (and how far away your plans are), it might be nice to pick up the phone and have a mini–catch-up before your real date. You have set aside this weekend for this purpose, so take advantage of it. There's truly nothing better than hearing a familiar voice on the other end of the phone. And a call, versus a text or an e-mail, speaks volumes (literally) about how much you care, especially in our frenetic digital age.

Don't worry if you have 10 people on your list to see and you have only one or two free time slots in the week. It's okay to make plans a few weeks or a month out. Remember, as busy as you are, it's likely your friends are, too. It may take coordination to find a time that works for both parties, but it will happen as long as you make the effort. Offering an option or two gives your friend some flexibil- ity, and if your proposals don't work, she will come back with another option. Eventually, you will find a time slot that suits you both.

**Follow up.** It's Saturday afternoon. While you're taking the initiative to sit down with your date book, not everyone you call will be sitting with her date book open as well. You will likely reach people who are out running around, or you may get voice mails. The easiest thing for you to do is to follow up the call with a text or an e-mail posing date options. (No one checks voice mail, or likes to, these days anyway!) This way, your friend can check her calendar at her leisure, with your available dates spelled out in front of her, and respond accordingly.

As you are reaching out and asking for plans, make one date for tomorrow. This can be coffee, brunch, a walk in the park, or anything that works for you and your friend. Since you have this weekend set aside, get started and make the first connection. You'd be surprised that as busy as everyone is, sometimes Sundays are left open-ended as the one day to relax and not commit to anything, and a last-minute plan can be a welcome surprise.

When you have worked through your list, tried everyone by phone, and then followed up with a text or an e-mail, you should feel great and really connected,

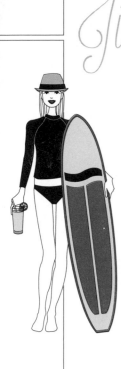

*Jill* I am not a huge birthday person. I admit I sometimes forget people's birthdays. But the good news is, I am all about making special days out of ordinary ones. I am known to knock on someone's door in the morning and kidnap him or her for a day of wild adventure. I don't need to have a full-out celebration on my birthday—I would much rather someone take me for an impromptu excursion!

*Dana* Every December, when I buy my new date book for the coming year (yes, I still use an actual paper date book), I transfer over birthdays. I sit there and write in everyone's day from January to the following December. This way, I am reminded of my friends' birthdays as they come up. For some reason, birthdays stick in my memory well (which is odd, because they are the only numbers I am good with), so the date book is my backup, but I think acknowledging a special day is an important and really easy way to show someone you care.

even if you haven't actually spoken to anyone yet! Your friends are the people who are there for you in good times and bad. They can relate to all that you are going through—whether work, relationship, family, or otherwise. It is superimportant for you to be available for your friends, just as you need them to be there for you. Relationships take care and nurturing, and you are on the road to doing that.

**Keep track of important anniversaries.** Still have your date book in front of you? Another great way to keep up with friendships is to enter all of your friends' birthdays (or at least those of close friends). A birthday is the one day of the year that is truly our own. It's not a family holiday or religious holiday or Hallmark holiday. You can easily make your friends feel special on that day by remembering to call, send a card, or, if you live in the same city, plan a celebration of some sort. Birthdays are great excuses to reconnect with people you have not seen or spoken to in ages.

A happy birthday wish is always welcome, especially coming from long-lost friends!

By now, you should feel emotionally full and rewarded. Hopefully, you have made a plan for tomorrow and set up other plans for the coming weeks. Don't worry if not everyone has responded with a date yet. They will. You've done a huge part just by making the effort to stay on top of the plan making.

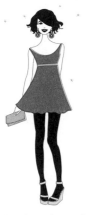

# SATURDAY NIGHT

If you already had a date with a friend set up for this evening (or if someone you asked for Sunday plans invited you out tonight instead), lucky you. If not, perhaps you have a favorite book or movie that reminds you of how much fun and how valuable girlfriends really are. You know the ones—the "chick flicks"—the ones that your boyfriend or husband sends you off with your girlfriends to watch while they are at the sports bar. Yeah, those. Take advantage of this opportunity to relive the tears and the giggles you had together and make a promise to not let those relationships slide any longer.

Enjoy your evening and look forward to reconnecting with your first friend tomorrow. If you don't have a Sunday plan yet in place, there's still time! If you hear back from anyone you reached out to who is available, lock in a time and place to meet tomorrow. Or try for one more reachout to someone you know is not great about checking their phone.

---

## 10 GREAT GIRLFRIEND MOVIES (OR CHICK FLICKS)

1. *Bridesmaids*
2. *Clueless*
3. *He's Just Not That into You*
4. *How to Make an American Quilt*
5. *Mystic Pizza*
6. *Romy and Michelle's High School Reunion*
7. *Sex and the City*
8. *Steel Magnolias*
9. *Thelma and Louise*
10. *Under the Tuscan Sun*

---

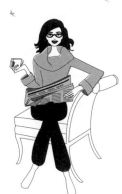

# SUNDAY

If yesterday you successfully made plans for today, fantastic! Enjoy your date with your girlfriend. Savor the time, even if it's just an hour, and try to schedule another date in the near future.

**Be spontaneous!** If you were not able to reach someone or make a definite plan for this afternoon, let's try again now. Yes, it is last minute, but you never know whether someone is available unless you try. Right? We sometimes jump to the conclusion that everyone else is just as busy, if not more so, than we are, so we rarely reach out and propose a last-minute, spontaneous get-together. But you'd be surprised how often you can find someone who is game and would love an impromptu catch-up with you.

Make a select round of calls and/or send a few texts to people who live close enough that you could realistically see them today. You can offer to stop by a friend's home if she is tied up with kids or whatnot and can't get away but has the time for a chat and a tea. At the very least, have a phone date with a friend who lives in another city if you are long overdue for a heart-to-heart. Do your best. If a plan doesn't coalesce, it's not the end of the world, but if it happens, great! Tip: If you reach out to enough people, likely someone will be around and available.

You have a second task today, in addition to your date: Go through your e-mails and texts again, follow up with anyone who responded to your initial outreach yesterday, and jot a date down in the book. Start filling your calendar with your upcoming plans. You'll also want to establish a system to manage friendships going forward so that you don't end up delinquent again. Here are suggestions:

**Commit to responding to calls, e-mails, and texts in a timely manner.** Whether that is at the end of every day; when you are done with work and before you head home to your man, kids, workout, or what have you; or first thing in the morning, before you get started with work or whatever else you have going on that day. If responding every day is unrealistic, commit to every other day, or set aside two or three times per week to do this. Maybe this is how you spend lunch breaks twice a week. Truly, whatever works for you is fine, as long as you do it.

**Dedicate one (or more) time(s) in your week or, at the very least, month, to see friends.** If a certain time slot works for you, strive to keep it filled with plans with different friends. For example, if you have a weekly lunch free, book a date with a different girlfriend in that time slot every week. Or make it a running date with the same girlfriend, and find other slots that work for other friends. Seeing your best friend every week—imagine that!

**Establish a set time to check and keep up with your friends list.** If you have the time on Sundays to take out your calendar and double-check that you have dates lined up, perfect. If it's not Sunday, pick another window that works for you and stick to it.

Well, you did it. You came back from the brink of obscurity and hopefully salvaged a few friendships along the way. You are now up to date with your correspondence and filled in on the latest goings-on of your friends and family. There are more rewarding moments to come as you continue to grow closer. Congrats and keep up the good work!

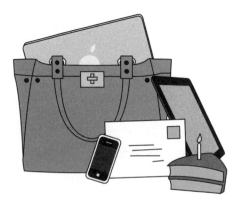

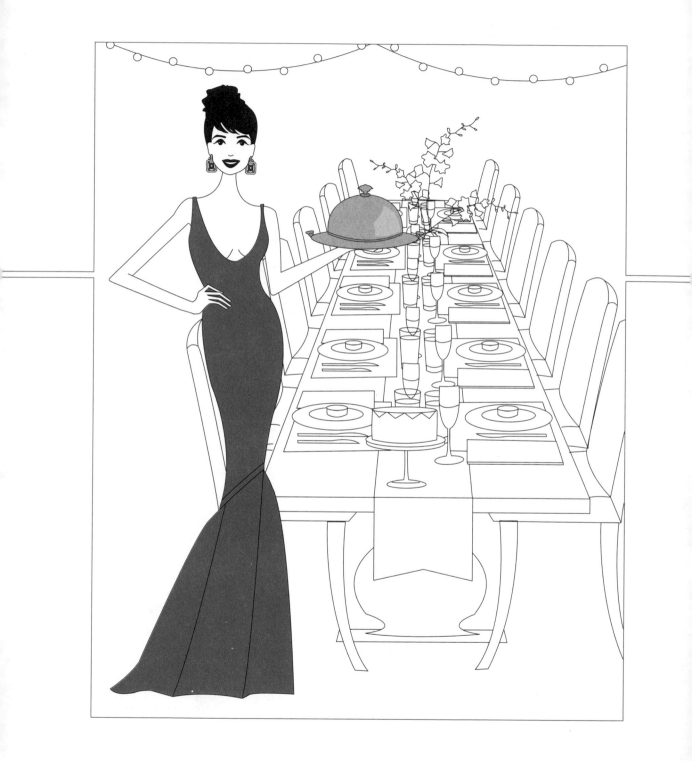

# Chapter Twelve
## Tradition Makeover

Do you dread the holidays or just about any family get-together? Are you stuck in a rut, doing the same thing year in and year out, and it's no longer fun? Do you find that the old family traditions aren't working for you anymore—or maybe they haven't worked since you were a kid?

Many family traditions were formed and set before you were born. When you were a child, you probably didn't have much say over how and where to spend Thanksgiving, Christmas, or July 4th. Maybe, just maybe, you got to decide how to celebrate your birthday. When we were young, these family get-togethers were often fun—you got to see your cousins, grandma and grandpa, and favorite aunt. These festivities pretty much consisted of playing, eating, and possibly opening presents.

As we get older, however, and establish our own lives and careers, form families of our own, and move away from home, we develop different ideas of what not only is fun but also is convenient and meaningful. The old traditions don't always fit this description, but somehow we feel trapped into celebrating the same way—or feel guilty if we don't.

This weekend, it's time for you to think about celebrating in a new manner. It doesn't matter if the celebration is for an actual holiday or if it is something special you want to start going forward—you're forging a new tradition, one that works for you. With a little research and planning, it's your turn to take charge and show everyone how it's done!

# 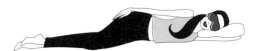 FRIDAY NIGHT

Your project for this evening is to think about your ideal celebration, gathering, or holiday. If you could start a new tradition, what would it be, where would it be, and who would attend?

Grandma or Cousin Sue or your own parents might have claim on certain holidays right now, and you don't want to ruffle feathers when you plan your own event. If you are happy with the circumstances surrounding your family celebrations, then maybe the tradition you start is not based on a holiday at all but is a random date that you choose to organize and host a get-together.

If you are not happy with the current state of the gatherings in your family, you can work to change it. Offer to host (instead of Cousin Sue). Or cohost, if lots of people are involved. You'll be surprised how quickly people may relinquish responsibility. It might not have occurred to them that there was another option, so they just kept chugging along with the way things were.

There are several reasons why the existing holidays may not be satisfying for you:

**Distance.** Perhaps you no longer live near most of your family, and it is a hassle and an expense for you to return home every Thanksgiving, Christmas, Hanukkah, Passover, Easter, or other holidays you celebrate.

**Travel.** If you don't live near the family home, traveling on and around the holidays is not much fun because of crowded highways, airports, train stations, etc. Year after year, the travel can get a bit much. Most long-distance holiday travel is done by car. The average long-distance trip is 214 miles at Thanksgiving and 275 miles over the Christmas/New Year's holiday. That's roughly 4-plus hours in the car one way!

**Lodging.** Again, if you don't live nearby, sleeping at relatives' homes—whether it means sharing a room or sleeping on the couch—can be uncomfortable when you don't have your own space. And hotels can be expensive.

**Food.** Most holidays are based around big meals and lots of eating. If you have been striving to eat healthier (see Chapter 1!), you might find it difficult to be surrounded by heavy foods and feel left out when the menu doesn't have anything suitable for you.

**Time off.** Having to take time off from work to accommodate travel may be an issue, especially if the holiday eats into your stock of vacation days that you'd rather use for a fabulous trip in summer.

**Family fights.** Aah, the biggest holiday stressor of all. We've all been in and around our families for so long (well, since we were born) that sometimes it seems as though we don't notice the drama any-

> ## 10 FAMILY GATHERING OPPORTUNITIES
>
> 1. Annual family reunion
> 2. Beach vacation
> 3. Career promotion
> 4. Celebration of sobriety
> 5. Child's birthday
> 6. Grandparents' anniversary
> 7. Housewarming
> 8. Picnic
> 9. Snow/ski holiday
> 10. Yearly 5k run

more. But truthfully, wouldn't it be so much nicer if there were less antagonism and if everyone spoke to each other civilly and got along? About three-quarters of those surveyed in a University of Connecticut poll said their family experiences conflict during holiday gatherings, and 28 percent said they are anxious about dealing with family conflicts. But of those who do experience conflict, half said they still want to connect with family, even if there are problems. So the point is to find a way to gather peacefully.

Taking on the role of host or cohost can alleviate a lot of what you find uncomfortable or inconvenient about these events. If you are capable of hosting one big family holiday yourself, think about making that your new tradition. If you want to cohost—meaning help plan, contribute input, and perhaps share some of the cost but not actually hold the event in your home—that's fine, too. Offer your help to

*Jill* *I love spending time with my family. My parents live half an hour away and my brother is closeby in the city. My mom and I speak all the time. Every Thursday when the Knicks are not playing, I take them to a new, cool restaurant, and we laugh the whole time. I feel so lucky to have them in my life.*

*Dana* *My grandmother is the matriarch of my family. She has been in charge since before I was born. (She just turned 93, and I am so lucky to still have her.) Her birthday has turned into one of our annual family gatherings. She lives in Florida, as does my sister and her family. I live in New York, and my parents are in North Carolina. For as long as I can remember, we have gathered in Gram's home for all the major holidays. Over the course of the 8 years I spent living in LA, this became a lot of travel for me. I ended up picking and choosing the holidays I would fly in for, and I decided to spend other holidays with cousins in San Diego or friends in LA.*

whoever is hosting now, or recruit a different family member and the two of you start from scratch.

**Start your own tradition.** If the big holidays are sorted, and everyone seems happy with the status quo, then plan something else. Maybe you want to have a giant celebration for your birthday each year, or maybe you would like an annual fun summer party since most of the big holidays are in the winter. Perhaps you could take on July 4th or another summer date to host a soiree.

By adding another get-together into the mix, you may decide to skip one or more other holidays that are difficult for you to attend. This way, you avoid the travel, time off, sleeping on the couch, and the food issues, and you still get to see your family! Even if you aren't hassled by holiday planning, you might just want to shake things up, and that's completely understandable. We sometimes forget that, as adults, we are not being told what to do by our parents anymore and that we have options.

The remedy to family issues? Well, that's a bit more complicated, but we will tell you that when nonrelatives are invited to a family event, it's amazing how quickly everyone gets on their best behavior. Think about inviting friends to your gathering as well as family. Friends who live far from home would love to celebrate a holiday locally, without having to travel themselves. Or perhaps you invite one close friend and his or her whole family as well, just to mix it up and all be together.

Decide what will work and be most realistic for you. If you live in a small apartment and don't have the capacity to host a large family dinner, take that into account. Instead, think about cohosting Thanksgiving with your sister or brother, if your sibling has the space. Another option is an outdoor party held in warmer weather at a park, a restaurant, or another venue.

Give real thought tonight to what you would like to be different and how you are going to change it. Pick the event/holiday/celebration that you are going to take charge of and start a new tradition for. Tomorrow, we'll start the actual planning.

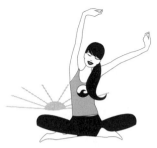

## SATURDAY MORNING

You should now know which holiday/gathering/party you are going to host or cohost. If you have chosen one of the major holidays, discuss your intention with the current host to ensure she or he, and everyone else in your family, is on board with the change. If you are starting a holiday from scratch, you should be good to go.

Now have breakfast, and then let's start organizing. . . .

*Jill* *I was never a fan of New Year's Eve. There's a lot of pressure to have a good time, especially when you're dating, and hats and noisemakers aren't my thing. So last year I started a new tradition and spent the holiday with dear friends, Stefani, Mitch and their adorable daughter, Theo. We ordered in Chinese food, watched the ball drop at midnight.....and the next morning I was the first at the gym. Good friends, good food, and a workout to start the new year..*

*Dana* *One year, when I was living in Miami near my family, I decided to go to Australia over the Thanksgiving holiday. Work was quiet for me that week, I had friends who invited me for a visit during their 3-month stay (a rare opportunity), and, since I am a raw vegan, the food at Thanksgiving is not really up my alley! My friends and I had our very own Thanksgiving celebration at a restaurant in Sydney, and we couldn't have been happier. That's what worked for me. Since I saw my family all the time anyway, I decided it was okay for me to skip the holiday this one year.*

**Make an invite list.** Once you have decided what and when you are going to host, the next step is to compile a list of guests. Is it going to be all of the usual suspects? Or do you want to reach wider and include family members who aren't normally in attendance? Or, better yet, do you want to combine family *and* friends?

Obviously, you weigh many considerations when deciding who to include. If you live near your family, then the only concern is the actual event. If you live farther afield, then travel and lodging are factors. Will everyone be game to stay in a hotel if need be? Are you willing to hold a smaller gathering if not everyone will want or be able to travel to you?

This is your shindig, so anything that sounds good to you and is viable sounds good to us! If only your immediate family wants to make the trip, fill up the empty seats at the dinner table with friends. If certain family members don't get along well, and this year you wish to eliminate the drama, keep the gathering small. Really, anything goes. Whatever your ideal scenario is (within reason), start to plan. You'll be amazed (or maybe not) how thrilled and relieved your friends will be to receive an invite to your holiday (even Thanksgiving or Christmas!) to avoid traveling or their own family dramas!

Now that you have sorted out your guest list, the event date, and the focus of the celebration, let's figure out what the event will entail and where it will be. Do you want the traditional sit-down meal around a big table, or would you rather the gathering be activity based? Will it be held during the day or in the evening? At your home, a restaurant, or some other venue? How much will it cost?

Some things to consider:

**Time of day.** If your gathering includes young kids and/or elderly members of your family, you may want to schedule your event during the day or in the afternoon or early evening.

**Activity.** If you include an activity in addition to or instead of a big meal, make sure everyone can participate. Before you decide to host your party at a bowling alley, think about the logistics of this for each guest. Playing board games or team-based charades at home is something that everyone can get involved with and enjoy.

**Food.** It seems these days that everyone has his or her own food specifications. Whether you are going to serve a formal meal or simply have snacks around, take food issues into account and offer something for everyone. You don't need to

## 6 FORMAL GATHERING IDEAS

1. Christmas morning breakfast
2. Cocktail party
3. Dinner and dancing at a country club
4. Elegant dinner at home
5. Professional family photo shoot
6. Upscale hotel restaurant brunch

serve "traditional" fare. Remember, you are starting your own tradition! Make it work for you and your guest list.

**Age.** You want everyone to be comfortable, so figuring out a setup that works for all ages involved is key. Having an activity to keep the kids occupied while the adults socialize is always smart. Finding activities that can include all age groups is even better.

**Venue.** Again, comfort is key, as is keeping costs down. Hosting at home may be economical. However, hosting at a restaurant may not always cost much more and would alleviate any cleanup and stress you might feel from having a crowd in your home. If your event is scheduled for one of the warmer months, a picnic in a nearby park can be an option that will both keep costs down and people out of your home!

*Jill*

*I have a few opinions when it comes to a budget for a party. Here is the deal: You do not have to spend a fortune to host a killer party. The best parties I have thrown involved mini-grilled cheese sandwiches, mini-hamburgers, french fries, pigs-in-a-blanket, and a Carvel "Fudgie the Whale" cake for dessert. You just have to create an environment that lets people have fun, dance, and let loose. Pick a fun theme, put on some good music, and choose simple food that everyone loves!*

*Dana*

*While I was living in LA, some friends and I created a tradition of our own. Every fall, three friends and I would host a breakfast. We invited everyone we knew! Who doesn't like a bagel? So many of us were from the East Coast and far from our own families. This was a fun, inexpensive, no-pressure way to have a celebration on our terms.*

**Budget.** Consider cost as you look into the above options. As we mentioned, a home-based event is generally (but not always) less expensive than one at a restaurant. A picnic can be very inexpensive. An activity with no meal involved might be very affordable. Take into account all of the costs, add them up, and see where you can compromise to make sure you are happy and comfortable with the results. A great idea is to cohost with another family member or even a friend and split the costs.

As you take into account all of the factors above, note that since you are starting a new tradition, you are also curating the whole experience. It is up to you to set the tone, the mood, and the vibe. You pick the dress code. Do you want to do it up and have everyone dress fancy, or do you prefer a more casual experience? You decide whether or not to have a theme and how to decorate the setting accordingly.

You need to take the initiative to make sure everyone is comfortable and having fun. If there is normally tension around family gatherings, look for a way to alleviate that. Have a list of conversation starters that will engage everyone and steer clear of uncomfortable, all-too-personal topics.

Lots of decisions, huh? As we mentioned, this is your gig, so do it your way. Of course, ask for any opinions or help from family or friends. It's good to get another opinion and some sound advice and help if you need it.

Once you have figured out what your ideal event will look like, take a little break. If you are hungry, have a nice lunch. Settle into your event choices (and have backup choices, just in case). This afternoon, we'll get on the computer and on the phone to start doing a little party research.

## 13 INFORMAL GATHERING IDEAS

1. Arts and crafts
2. Beach day/pool party
3. Board games/charades
4. Boating
5. Bowling
6. Cookie decorating
7. Hors d'oeuvres and the Big Game on TV
8. Karaoke
9. Miniature golf
10. Picnic/field games
11. Pumpkin carving
12. Scavenger hunt
13. Volunteering at a soup kitchen

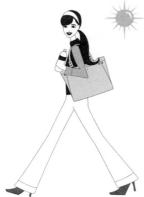

# SATURDAY AFTERNOON

Take time now to map out the logistics. If you are considering a restaurant, explore your choices and the costs involved. How many people can the restaurant accommodate? What is the menu, and is it prix fixe or à la carte? If you are considering hosting a meal at home, check with restaurants or catering companies for cost estimates for your number of guests. If you will cook yourself, the meal will likely be less expensive but could be very labor intensive, depending on what you plan to serve. Note how much seating you have at home and whether you will need or want to rent or borrow tables and chairs or if you wish to keep it casual and buffet-style with people perched around the living room, etc.

If you hold an outdoor gathering at a park or beach, for example, check into the rules or policies at those public venues so you know how to prepare, what to expect, what it will cost (if anything), and whether you need to reserve or get a permit. Consider what else you will need at outdoor venues—blankets, towels, food, etc.

Same goes for any other activity—whether it's bowling, playing miniature golf, or celebrating at a karaoke bar. Gather all the details to properly plan and reserve a time and place. Can you get a group rate? What other food or amenities are offered? Interactive activities are great for breaking the ice and releasing any family tensions that might normally be present—a big plus!

**Book it!** Once you have decided on the venue, whether the event will feature a meal or an activity, the event time and date, and the number of expected guests, set it in stone. Or at least reserve the event space. For an event held outside of your home, another bit of information you will need is whether a deposit is required and, if so, if it is refundable.

Inviting a large number of people? Then you will want to reserve the location far in advance, especially before you invite people who must make travel arrangements to attend. Even if your event is a small party, you don't want to mess with

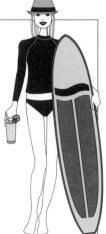

*Jill* I work 6 or 7 days a week, so I need help whenever I am planning a party at my home. If I am going to splurge on one thing, it will be to hire someone to help clean and to manage the dishes and courses throughout the night. For me, there is nothing worse than having disarray at a party and/or a big mess at the end of the night.

*Dana* When I lived in LA, one summer I had my birthday party on the beach in Malibu. My cousin Victoria helped me organize it. We did a little research online, picked a great spot at one of the public beaches that everyone could find on the map, brought a couple of coolers with drinks and food from a little taco/burrito place, set up balloons so everyone invited could find us, and had ourselves a beach day. Even the invite was beachy—with a picture of a beach ball, a palm tree, sand, and the ocean. It was probably one of my favorite birthday celebrations. It did not turn into a tradition per se, but I do try to come up with fun and different ways to celebrate my birthday every year, depending on where I am living.

the time and date that you've set your heart on, so lock in the venue before you do the inviting.

**Plan the meal ahead of time.** Whenever a formal meal is involved, square the menu with the restaurant or caterer well in advance (especially if the event occurs around a traditional holiday when other people will be ordering, too). If you are doing the cooking yourself, obviously, you can wait until the week of to do the grocery shopping, but plan the menu now.

Once you have the meal planned, you can think about decorating, flowers, candles, party favors, or anything else you want to incorporate.

You now have all the fixings to start a new tradition! Like all traditions, it just starts with one great event that will make everyone want to celebrate again the same way next year.

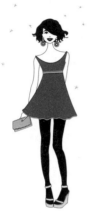

# SATURDAY NIGHT

Since this is your weekend to start a brand-new tradition (or, at the very least, to revamp and update the same old family gathering), take advantage of this time and do it right. Think of it is as research for your tradition makeover project. Get some trusted and festive friends involved and go for a "test drive" tonight. This is it—your opportunity for a trial run! Make it a mini-event, a rehearsal, before you commit to hosting the actual "big" event.

If you intend to host your holiday or party at a restaurant, try out the eatery tonight—on a smaller scale, of course. If you desire to host and cook a dinner for 12, tonight cook a full meal for two or, better yet, four, to see if you are up for meal preparation on a larger scale.

If you plan to host a bowling party or something of that nature, check out the venue tonight with a friend or your husband. Recruit a fun group for karaoke or find a foursome for miniature golf. Try to get a sense if this is something everyone on your list would enjoy—including you! Getting feedback might help you decide "yay" or "nay" to the venue, the activity, or all of the above.

Keep in mind that it is a very different prospect to "host" an event, especially an organized activity, outside the home than it is to entertain guests in your living space. There's no right or wrong here. We're just saying, try to get a feel for whether or not you are going to be up for a major holiday, meal-type event at your dining table, or if you'd rather keep it supereasy, activity oriented, and definitely not at home.

If you have your heart set on going the traditional route by taking over hosting duties for an existing holiday celebration—fantastic. If not, maybe you and your pals can spend a little time this evening brainstorming some creative ideas, reasons, excuses to have a party—not that you need one! And if you want to get really inventive, you can even prepare and practice giving a toast to welcome and thank your guests for their attendance. Cheers!

Have fun, take notes on the details, and tonight, just sleep on it. Make sure you are thrilled with your choice before the invites go out and while you can still change your mind!

## TOP **10** TOASTS

1. Congratulations on new baby
2. Congratulations on new job
3. Congratulations on new marriage/anniversary
4. Good health
5. Good luck
6. Happy birthday
7. Happy holidays
8. Happy new year
9. Thank you to the guests
10. Thank you to the host/hostess

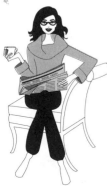

## SUNDAY

If you are happy with all of your decisions—time, date, venue, menu, activity, theme, dress code, and invite list— and have managed to keep the costs within your budget, congratulations! This is a huge accomplishment, and oh-so-very adult of you.

**Let everyone know.** With everything set, it's time to send out the invites (or at least a save-the-date card)! If you'd like to go the traditional route, written or printed invitations are always lovely. These days, however, it is perfectly acceptable and appropriate (not to mention faster and cheaper) to send out an e-mail invite through online sites like Evite.com or PaperlessPost.com.

Pick an invitation that represents whatever theme you are choosing for your party/dinner/celebration. Remember to list all the necessary info on the invite.

## 8 FAVE CUSTOM PRINT INVITE SITES

1. Erincondren.com
2. Etsy.com
3. Minted.com
4. Papyrusonline.com
5. Purpletrail.com
6. Shutterfly.com
7. Thestationarystudio.com
8. Tinyprints.com

Then, get your e-mail list together, take a deep breath, and hit Send!

You did it! Well, you planned it, anyway. We're sure the actual event will be a huge success—enough so that you and everyone else will want to celebrate your new tradition for years to come. Now that the invites are out, the ball is in motion and you must keep up with the RSVPs and all of the other details. If the head count changes, be sure to alert the venue (if you are hosting outside the home).

Block out time and dates in your calendar to take care of details that are best addressed closer to the actual event—food shopping and securing decorations, flowers, party favors, candles, and table and chair rentals. Give yourself enough time so that this event is a fun and pleasant experience you will want to host again and again. Recruit whatever help you want or need. Remember, this is a celebration on your terms, with your family and your friends. This is a good thing!

The even better thing is that once you have done the research and preparation entailed in hosting this new tradition, restaging the event gets easier and easier with each passing year. Now that you have laid the groundwork, next year all you need to do is rebook or redo it!

If your event is the huge success that we know it will be, take the initiative to organize it again for the following year as soon as you have rested from this year's splendid event. Enjoy!

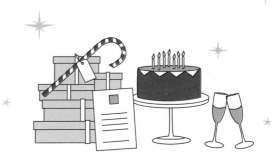

*Jill* *My mother and father host Thanksgiving. It is their* favorite
*holiday to host. My mom doesn't cook (although when she reads this,*
*she'll say, "Yes, I do!"). What my parents do well is* produce a party.
*They cater everything except the turkeys, which my dad cooks*
*(one in the oven, one on the grill), display dinner perfectly, and make*
*sure there is something for everyone. In my family we have a vegan,*
*a diabetic, and a cousin who is extremely picky!*

*Dana* *As my grandmother has gotten older, and it has*
*become more stressful for her to host big holidays in her home, we*
*have changed our tradition. We now celebrate all big family gatherings*
*at my sister's. We keep the activities mellow for Gram and my*
*younger niece and nephew. I consider myself a cohost, as I help my*
*sis with the logistics and planning, especially the menu. My*
*grandmother is no longer in charge of that department! We have*
*found more creative and healthier menus so there's something*
*for everyone—including me!*

# Congrats! You did it!

You have taken the initiative, invested the time, and successfully completed a makeover—hopefully one, two, or even all twelve of them. In essence, you have done much more than organize your closet or plan a vacation. You've created a whole new life for yourself—a full, healthy, beautiful, and more relaxed existence. You deserve it and hopefully you feel confident, happy, and rewarded. You should be very proud.

However, we all know that life can throw us curve balls. Sometimes things happen that can temporarily take us off of our path. People move, change jobs, have a baby (or a second or third), and our routines can get shifted. Don't let these things knock you off your game or let them keep you from your goal.

The same goes for traveling or anytime our lives get particularly hectic. We know all too well the temptation to eat junk, get lazy about working out, or letting our apartments pile up with laundry. But you don't have to throw everything you have established to the wind. No matter where you are, you can find something healthy to eat (or you can pack snacks with you), go for a long walk, read a book or study on the plane, and take care of your skin. All it takes is a little extra planning to make sure you have what you need.

If you get momentarily sidetracked from your new routine, take a deep breath and commit to getting back on track. Go back through this book for inspiration, reread the chapters you need to, and start again. Since you already know the drill, it might take just one day (not the whole weekend) to get yourself righted. Go to one workout class or choose to eat one healthy meal, and you are back in the game! It's that easy.

You are worth the time and effort to plan for your very own success, so no matter the circumstances, make it happen! We are so proud of you. Live, love, breathe, and have fun!

# ACKNOWLEDGMENTS

A huge "thank you" to:

David Zinczenko and Stephen Perrine for their wisdom, support, and foresight.

Ursula Cary, Christina Gaugler, Nancy Bailey, Sara Vigneri, Danielle Lynn, Brent Gallenberger, and the rest of the team at Rodale for their attention, skill, and creativity.

Mel Berger, Strand Conover, Evan Warner, Mark Mullett, and Henry Reisch at WME for their knowledge, advice, and guidance.

Sarah Hall, Lisamarie Gina, Julie Chudow, Danielle Burch, Kelly Wolf and Jenna Guarneri at Sarah Hall Public Relations for their dedication, imagination, and resourcefulness.

Natalie Morales, Dwyane Wade, and Adam Glassman for their time, generosity, and fabulousness.